I0704125

Tummy Story

Digestion in the Age of Processed Foods
and Antibiotics

Revised Edition

The Lay Health Detective's Manual

Patricia Mitchell Lapidus

Introduction to the Revised Edition

When I published *Tummy Story* in 2017 I expected that others with digestive problems would take an interest, and that did happen. As well, quite a few used the book as a guide for where to look for help with their own longstanding issues brought on by overuse of antibiotics and our modern diet. What surprised me was the number of readers who valued the book because it touched on the history of allopathic medicine and how other treatment methods were deliberately edged out. Some mentioned the history of farming and how our family farms, including my father's farm, have been mostly lost *in parallel to our lost health.*

Since the book had a wider appeal than I expected, I've decided to put out a second edition that emphasizes those parts of our history. Knowledge is power. I hope this edition will give you the information you need to rebuild your health and support those health practitioners who help people heal themselves and stay healthy.

My personal story continues to be a triumph against all odds. I've managed a troubled body into several further years of happy living. By the end of the first edition I had discovered the roots of my troubles way back in infancy. Since then those lines of family and personal history have sharpened into sure knowledge. It's fun, really fun, to know what happened. I look back at the times I was not able to do what others could do and I go, Ahah, there's another incident explained.

I knew I wasn't going to pull this elder body completely out of trouble. To do that I'd have to go back to my mother's health before I was conceived. In short, I'd have to start with a different body. But I wouldn't choose any different life from the one I've known. I love my story as it has unfolded. Most of us do prefer out own stories.

My days are busy. I work hard hour by hour at keeping my health up. If I gave you a list of the motions I go through each morning by the time I put my first meal on the table, you would find just reading the list exhausting. I know very few people for whom a big breakfast that includes vegetables is crucial and must be eaten within an hour of rising. But I'm not complaining. These are the terms by which I live, and the living is, as my Maine childhood prompts me to say, wicked good.

Introduction to the First Edition

The Home Health Spa, 2012 to 2017. From time to time when my illnesses threatened to get the best of me, I dreamed of going someplace where I would be fed the best diet, given optimum care, and coached at exercise. But even if I could find such a place, it would cost too much. If I wanted to live, I had to provide what I needed. In 2012 when I moved into the hills, I became my own chef, meal planner, and health researcher, coordinating the guidance of doctors from several disciplines and the few internet sources I trusted. By the fall of 2017 my program had cured both Candida and hypothyroidism. Leaky gut was a thing of the past. With help, the program I set for myself had discovered and tamed a bacterial pathogen going back years. My program had prescribed an exercise routine to protect thinning bones, keeping muscles strong and active to prevent falls. Organs were happier, as was the endocrine system. Dangerously low potassium and salt had been remedied with supplements. And that's the short list. It was either find answers or let go of this body and start over.

I took up the study of health because I was forced to do it. As for the answers I found, I don't know that I can explain everything—I'm not a medical professional—but I have discovered much that I wish I had known years earlier. I'm laying my discoveries out for others who are looking for answers and not finding them. The wisdom gained from soothing and healing one unhappy body belongs to all.

We have knowledge and resources now that were not available to me when I was younger. These days, medical doctors often combine their scientific training with older approaches to healing.   Alternative Medicine has made a comeback.   The internet offers a wealth of information as long as you are careful. Learning what resources to trust is a gradual process best taken a step at a time. The key question with any treatment is, "Does it work?"

It was only while writing the book that I and my doctors put my deep health history together well enough for a robust treatment plan.

Though treatments here may not be for everyone, the method I used is widely applicable. Research, finding doctors, talking with friends, and, best you can, buying food grown in, or pastured on, local nutrient-rich soil free of chemicals and pesticides. Above all, make your home into a health spa for one patient, you. Then,

1) Pay attention to your body.
2) Find and evaluate resources.
3) Consult health practitioners you trust.

A Word about Trust. Trust is both necessary to survival and problematic. You don't want to trust only to find yourself poorly served or betrayed. And yet, to trust no one is to limit both your pleasure in life and your survival.

I needed to trust the health practitioners in this account, at least provisionally. But I was not called upon to trust any of them absolutely. Any time I saw signs of incompetence, lack of compassion, or a stubborn belief that their training represented the only way, I could withdraw my trust and look elsewhere.

My doctors were recommended by friends I'd known for years, friends who had been healed or kept healthy by these healers.

Can you trust the internet? With caution. One can find a lot of useful information on the net. But don't follow the guidance of strangers without careful inspection and consultations with people you know and trust. And keep in mind that a negative articles about a method or doctor could be planted by Big Money. The status quo is like the fox in the story *Chicken Little,* offering to show us the way to the king but leading us into its den. Perhaps you have had reason to discover the lengths to which some of the big players will go to discredit honest healers.

The caution about trust applies to me, too. Don't trust anything I say in this book unless you find it true.

How about trusting ourselves? I don't know about you, but I was taught not to trust my experiences and perceptions. I was taught to override my observations and to believe instead a parent's line or a cultural "truth." In order to heal myself, I had to rehabilitate my ability to observe and trust what I observed. Little by little I learned to know what my body was telling me and to use the best treatments. Remember: the only test of a treatment is, does it work?

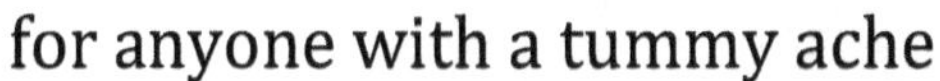

for anyone with a tummy ache

Contents

Tummy Story

2017. I am 75 years old. I stand straight and walk briskly. I live independently, spend time with grandchildren, and write. Such longevity and quality of life are a surprise.
I expected to die young.

What to Feed a Baby, 1942. A six-weeks-old infant lies in a baby carriage in the family's kitchen. Born underweight, she is hungry. For the last hour she has been crying in an insistent high-pitched scream. Her arms and legs beat back and forth, drumming her distress. She has kicked out of the swaddling blanket.

The baby's big sister toddles from the carriage across the kitchen to grab their mother's skirt where she stands washing dishes. The baby pulls on the skirt and says, "Ow!" It is one of her few words.

"I know, Winky," the mother says. "Trishy is hungry. But she's hungry all the time. If I nurse her now I won't have supper ready for your father."

Winky looks up at her mother with wide brown eyes as if she understands. She toddles back to pat the carriage. If she could talk she would tell Trishy not to cry.

The infant cries more urgently.

"I've had enough of this!" the mother says, drying her hands on a dish towel. "You go on a bottle." She sets a pan of water on the wood cook stove in which she has built a fire for baking biscuits. She gets a pitcher from the ice box in the shed and pours milk into a small-necked baby bottle, adding a dollop of clear Karo syrup from a bottle she sets back into the cupboard. This is the formula the doctor recommended for Winky when she stopped breastfeeding her at almost four months. She pulls a rubber nipple on over the neck of the bottle and into the groove below the rim. She bends the top of the nipple to keep the mixture from spilling and shakes the contents. Pulling the pan of water off the heat, she puts the bottle in the water, leaning it at an angle to get most of it into the warm water.

Suddenly all is quiet in the kitchen. The infant, worn out from crying, has fallen asleep. Winky can be heard playing under the window, putting a block on top of another with a small click, talking to the blocks in sweet baby sounds.

The mother sets ingredients on the counter, mixes and spoons biscuits into a pan and slides the pan into the oven box, her motions quick and efficient. She slips out to the ice box and takes out yesterday's roast chicken. The green beans on the stove will round out the meal.

Mercifully, the infant sleeps through supper. When she wakes, the mother takes her into the bedroom for a diaper change. Coming back out with the little girl on her shoulder, she takes the bottle from the pan and manages to test a drop of milk on the wrist of the arm that holds the baby. She sits down in the rocking chair and offers the bottle to the baby, who, after a taste of the sweet milk, begins to suck. The baby takes a full three ounces and sleeps again, this time for several hours.

The infant survived to tell the story. With quite a will, too. When I was six months old Mom found me creeping down the gravel path, having gotten myself down some shallow steps. I had scraped my tummy raw and had not cried. I was heading out.

I know the bottle story because it was often told to me. "You were born skinny and you screamed for six weeks. When I gave you cow's milk with Karo syrup, you shut up."

I never did think to apologize.

2017. I recently bought some seaweed salad from the Asian food vendor in our local market. It looked harmless, shredded seaweed and a little oil. In the leisure of my home, with reading glasses, I found there were seventeen ingredients, including sugar and two food dyes. Yikes!

Food and Family Life, 1940s. In the decade when my personal life began, families all over America were still making a living on farms. These were the war years. Dad volunteered but he was told to stay on the farm and grow food. Birth control was unknown, especially among farmers and working class people. My parents had seven children within a decade. They were delighted. Farmers needed a crew to tend the farm. By age seven, children carried buckets of grain. They tramped the loose hay the farmer pitched onto the pickup, firming the load for the trip to the barn and into the upper mow. They helped sow and hoe and reap. A young child could handle a draft horse—until the farmer switched over completely to the Farmall tractor that now sat in the barn. Inside, children swept floors, washed dishes, and carried trash out to the incinerator barrel. They learned to cook and bake and sew.

Food was mostly homegrown vegetables and meat. Meanwhile, small markets in town carried flour and other staples—salt, sugar, molasses, baking powder, vinegar for canning, a few spices. There was nothing like a supermarket or a mall. You shopped for clothing from the Sears & Roebuck catalogue or you drove to the nearest city where department stores were part of a thriving Main Street.

White refined sugar, or processed sugar as we know it today, was a new offering, one we accepted without thought. We sprinkled a spoonful of it on our morning Cheerios, Rice Krispies, or Cornflakes. Dad liked pillow-shaped Shredded Wheat; one pillow filled up his bowl and he sprinkled it with sugar before pouring on milk which he himself had milked from the cow, strained, and set to cool in the refrigerator. When I was twenty-four, a doctor told me maybe refined sugar wasn't good for people. I thought, *but sugar is food.* There seemed to be no slot in my mind for *sugar as problem.*

It would be many more years before anyone questioned eating processed cereals or, finally, grain itself, especially grain grown with glyphosate (Roundup).

The Curious History of a Tummy, 1948. I really shouldn't be here. How did I live through this one?   At 20 months – my mother was overdue to give birth to my sister Meddy – I toddled outside, got down some steps, and played in the gravel driveway. The hired man didn't see me. He backed over me, crushing my head between a back wheel and the gravel. I had gravel embedded in one cheek, tire treads deep in the other. I cried for three days at my grandmother's house while Mom went to the hospital to give birth.   Must have had a headache. But for that loose gravel, I wouldn't be here. See what I mean about miracles?

The down slope. Thanksgiving Day when I was six, Grammie and Mom and the aunts were checking the ovens, making gravy, stirring butter into bowls of winter squash, setting out pies. I wandered through the living room where the long table was set for the meal and climbed the stairs, thinking perhaps I would lie down in the familiar room where I sometimes stayed. Feeling too sick to lie down, I wandered back downstairs and into the kitchen. I could not tell my mother I was sick, not on Thanksgiving Day when she was happy and visiting. So I drifted back upstairs and down again in a hopeless repetition.

I have never forgotten that feeling, one unlike any other. Knowing that distinct feeling would come in handy many years later when I had learned to identify it as toxicity.

I don't remember how I got through that long ago Thanksgiving dinner. Hard to believe I ate anything. Only the pain stands out in memory.

Back home I sat on the couch while the family moved around me. Four days before Christmas my grandmother came to visit. She took one look at me and told my mother to take me to the doctor. The doctor looked at my hands where he found scaling, evidence that I had had scarlet fever. He said, "Most children get through scarlet fever okay, but in a few it goes into a secondary infection that is bacterial. Do you want to take her to the hospital this afternoon or tomorrow?" Mom drove me the seven miles to the hospital that afternoon. The doctor gave me a fifty-fifty chance.

Settled in a big white bed in a white room with nurses coming and going in white dresses and white caps and white stockings and white shoes, I got the first of many penicillin shots. The nurse had me turn over, took a handful of my bottom, and pushed the needle in. I was too sick to care about the sting.

My system was toxic because my kidneys, under attack from rogue bacteria, were shutting down. The little glomeruli that sift the blood, instead of sending purified blood back into circulation, were cycling blood back without cleaning—and losing blood in the urine. I remember brown pee.

After a couple of weeks the infection was gone and my pee was yellow. Sometime in January I went home to recuperate on bed rest and salt-free meals my mother brought upstairs to my crib. Yep. I was in a crib to keep me from getting up and because the crib was in my parents' bedroom where Mom could keep an eye on me. She was cheerful about the many trips up and down stairs. My mother often whistled while she worked.

What I experienced after recovery and for the rest of my days is relevant to the health struggles of large numbers of people whose lives were saved by antibiotics long before anyone understood what would happen to our tummies. That is the downward slope. My caretakers read my slumps as if the kidneys had not completely healed. They put me to bed for rest a couple times a year. They did not know that penicillin would wreck my tummy ecology—and never guessed another hidden problem.

2017. After I pull up the blinds each morning, I turn on the computer. When I'm in the middle of writing a book, I need the manuscript handy in case I think of something to include. As well, I keep in touch with family and friends via email and facebook.

Communications, Pharmaceuticals, and Culture, 1948 to 1958. To show the general state of living in those days, I'll give a few examples. We had a crank telephone on the kitchen wall. You picked up the earpiece, which was tethered to the phone by a short cord. You rang the operator by use of a crank and spoke into the wall phone, telling the operator the home you wanted to reach. After a pause, she connected you.

We had a party line and only used the phone for farm business or something as urgent as calling the doctor. Our social life we pursued at church, at family gatherings, or in school. Remembering those phones and talking about social networking today, someone quipped that some inadvertent networking went over those party lines. Some neighbors listened in and, anyway, you heard all sorts of things when you picked up to speak with the operator.

As you look at the picture, notice the two eyes. Those are the bells that alerted us of an incoming call. Directly below is the speaker. If you were short you had to stand on tip-toe to reach it. On the left is the earpiece cradled in metal arms. And on the right is the crank, almost invisible. I remember watching Mom put the earpiece to her ear, wind the crank a few times, and wait for the operator.

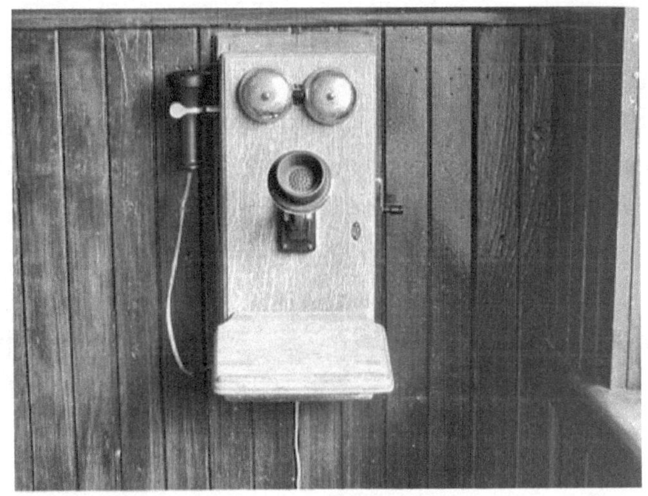

We had radios, one in the house and another in the egg room where Dad listened to comedies and stories—*Our Miss Brooks, Jack Benny, The Lone Ranger, The Shadow.* ("Who knows what evil LURKS in the hearts of men? The Shadow knows.") Baseball. Dad cleaned the eggs and set them to roll onto the grader. While I put graded eggs into cases, he explained how Lou Boudreau should manage the Red Sox.

Chemical pharmaceuticals, though not new, surged into common use after the war. The Rockefellers gave large amounts of money to medical colleges on condition that only pharmaceutical treatments be taught. (See YouTube documentary *The Rockefellers Exposed*.) This was to ensure that the new drug companies they owned, creating products based on petroleum, would prosper.

My grandfather knew all the plants in the fields and forests, their names and uses. He didn't pass this knowledge down to his children and grandchildren. We didn't know we would one day wish we had learned it. People were happy to let the drug companies decide and provide. Not very responsible of us. In the beginning the new drugs didn't cost much and were far fewer than the array of prescriptions a pharmacist dispenses today.

My mother's medicine chest contained aspirin, Band-aids, Vaseline, and topical antiseptics such as Mercurochrome and Iodine.

As for the social culture in the 1950s, we in Yankee Maine believed democracy in the United States was working, simple and above board. We had no inkling that some of the activities of humankind had compromised the earth's ecology, much less climate. Most families lived on one income. Mothers stayed home, did the housework and cooking, and were there to greet children coming home from school.

Our family sat down to meals together. We set the table while chanting a little rhyme: *bread and butter, salt and pepper, knives, forks, spoons, plates, and tumblers*. The plates were blue or green pastel Melmac wear and the tumblers were metal painted different colors on the outside, a subdued yellow, pink, green, blue. I can see them still. The noon meal was called dinner and consisted of meat, potatoes, and vegetables, bread on the side. After my illness, when I needed bread without salt, Mom learned to make bread.

We ate store bread as well. One afternoon during my teens, a friend and I were leaving the house when my father came to the door with some fifteen loaves of day-old Wonder Bread stacked on his arm. My friend quipped, "Here comes the breadwinner."

The lighter evening meal was called supper, from the word *soup*. Farmers worked hard and needed plenty of food for breakfast and dinner; after supper they didn't expect to be heading out to do haying and such.

We kept a set of encyclopedias near the table to address questions that came up during the meal. Together with a Webster's Dictionary, these sufficed for all inquiries.

Our winter entertainments were many. We had card games such as Go Fish and Old Maid. We had Parcheesi and Clue. We played checkers and caroms. I recall many a happy hour putting a puzzle together, the whole family gathered round, teasing and laughing and contributing to the project. I remember some of the pictures and even the way the pieces felt. We still do puzzles when we get together.

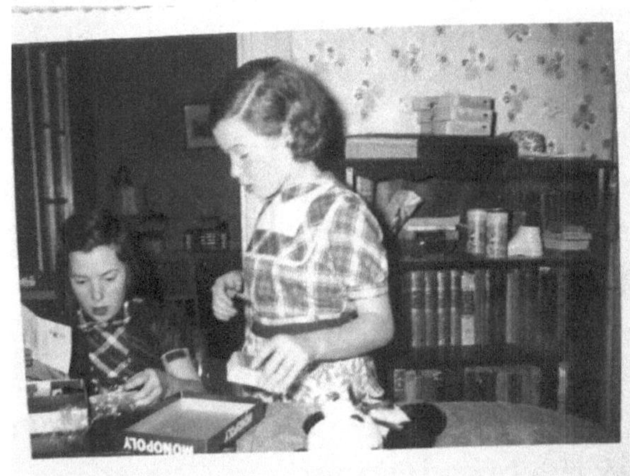

One Christmas we got Monopoly. In the picture I'm studying the directions while Winky holds the cards that tell you what to do. (It was from Monopoly cards that a now familiar saying came into common use. "Go directly to jail. Do not pass GO. Do not collect $200.")

These days very few people grow up on farms, but almost all of us have grandparents or great-grandparents who did spend their early years on farms, eating good farm food, doing chores that kept them fit, and roaming the fields and woods, maybe fishing in brooks or hunting deer. It's back there a generation or more in our genes and in the stories we heard when we were young. Those farms protected our health, until they didn't.

2021 note, included on the urging of my friend Dr. Robin Rose: With the growth of industrial farming on a huge scale, some very dangerous chemicals and technologies came into use. One of the worst is the spraying of Roundup. Roundup contains glyphosate, a chemical that erodes the gut lining, causes leaky gut, and destroys our tender mitochondria, the tiny filaments that do the work of taking up and using nutrients. But I'm not a chemist and even after listening and reading about this I'm not the person to explain it. You can look up Dr. Alex Vasquez or research the effects of glyphosate. And while you do that, look up what Genetically Modified Foods do to our systems. I avoid GMOs and most American grains because these two demon problems have spread from the fields where they started and contaminated most American soil.

2017. My table is cluttered with books. Some are about food, digestion, and metabolism. Sometimes I take a book with me to the exer-bike. I spin while I read. This morning I re-read a passage in Dr. Eric Berg's book The Seven Principles of Fat Burning. *It's a controversial title. An alternative doctor I trust doesn't agree. But Berg makes sense to me. Fat is my fuel.*

The Curious History of a Tummy Continues, 1950s. Emotional stress may be a factor in anyone's health story. My parents, although kind and generous, brought forward from their own childhoods the authoritarian ways of Maine Yankees. Easily upset by the antics of children, my mother believed the bad basic nature of her children had to be spanked out of them. (When another mother commented that she didn't spank her children because she "didn't want to warp their little natural dispositions," Mom's response was that some children needed their little natural dispositions warped.)

Being spanked hard and long made me feel thrown away. It didn't teach me anything except that I was a disappointment. In a well-researched book *Raised by Animals: The Surprising New Science of Animal Family Dynamics* (2017), Jennifer L. Verdolin reports many similarities between human and animal family interactions, but one thing she does not find among animals is hitting the young as a means of training. What she finds instead is animal parents gently insisting. Further, most animal babies and children sleep with their parents for safety and warmth and comfort. She found parents and others cuddling babies and carrying them around a lot.

No doubt I was a cute child, but few babies could aspire to the standard of cuteness set by my older sister. In recent years I asked our father, "Was Winky a cute baby?" He said, "Oh, was she cute!" He told of a time they had taken her out to a Grange meeting in a long white dress "with her little shoes peeking out."

While my sister was a helper child, I was carefree. My high spirits drew spankings. Whatever the reason, and no matter how much I empathize now with my mother, my conflicts with her in infancy and as a toddler were detrimental to my confidence. Confidence is, after all, nothing more or less than a person's self. Feeling pushed away made me vulnerable to illness. I have little doubt of that. Since many parents in today's broken culture are as uninformed about punishment and the need for comfort as my parents were, we can note that much childhood illness follows along the lines mine did. *Your tummy could be hurting because your heart is hurting.*

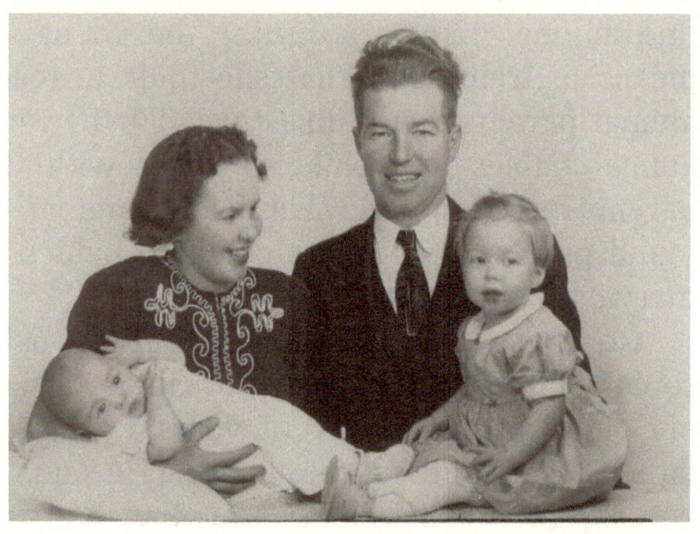

Lucky for me, Grampa and I were best pals from the start. I'd crawl to meet him and he would gather me up and say, "Grampa's girl." I saw my grandparents often. But when I was five we moved to a different farm some fifteen miles distant, making visits infrequent. Perhaps it is no coincidence that I got sick soon after the move. Along with missing Grammie and Grampa, I missed the ancestral hill farm where I was born, its nooks and smells, the view from the orchard hill. It was an emotional loss for

Dad, as well, but the new farm was better for business.

Among the people I've talked to about modern life, many have known losses that impacted their health and happiness. We are a nation of movers, and we often lose beloved relatives as well as homes and friends and neighborhoods.

Still, kids are resilient. I had the new farm and woods to roam. There was hay to jump in, a swing to pump high, and trips to swim at Grampa's pond or off the ledges at Orr's Island. There were family camping trips and hikes along the shore to where waves made smooth the ledges and the rocks that beat against them.

But much as I loved our outings, I often lacked the energy to fully enjoy them. Once on a mountain hike we met a woman who took several strides down a side trail, realized her mistake, and reversed in several more quick strides to the juncture she had missed. My father said, "Some women are remarkably able." There was no comparing my energy to hers.

I was often too tired to go to school the week before Christmas or the week before the school picnic in June. Mom assumed my kidneys were at fault. She noticed dark circles under my eyes and put me to bed. Even when I was relatively well, my tummy was round with distress. Mom would admonish me, "Pull in your tummy." As if I could. I doubt it ever occurred to her to relate my distended belly to the earlier illness and antibiotics or to see it as a sign of trouble. She didn't know to think like that.

There was much fussing over me, worry that my kidney troubles would flare up. I thought I was not expected to live to grow up. I'd lie in bed at night wondering if the very next instant was the one when I would die. I guess I became a bit wimpy.

My mother decided my attitude needed to change. She showed me a picture of a bird with peering eyes in *The Ladies Home Journal.* "This is a watch bird watching a helpless hopeless. Are you a helpless hopeless?" Mom told me, "This is you." And it well may have been true. My lack of energy was real, but I was also discouraged. Of course, the criticism only sank me deeper. I believed I was a helpless hopeless.

By high school I stopped missing school and enjoyed my studies. I did my share of morning chores, feeding calves and chickens. After homework I graded or gathered eggs, filling several wire baskets with eggs from nests along the walls of the pens and loading the baskets onto the open elevator for a trip down to the egg room.

In late October we brought chickens in off the range. After dark, Dad drove out with the pickup and a crew of three or four of his kids. By then the birds had settled in the shelters and were sleepy, easy to pick up. Dad would crawl in first and start passing them out by the legs. One of us would sit at the shelter door to pass chickens on to the next person in line where they were either crated or thrown into the truck, depending on which floor of the henhouse they were destined for. If it was the first floor we could put them into the truck loose and toss them in through a window. For the second floor we children stood by while Dad launched each pullet and young rooster into flight through an upper window. The crated hens for the third floor went up the elevator, an open conveyance with a rope pull.

On trips to the range for the next batch of chickens we took time to enjoy the night sky and learn the constellations. We joked and teased and became a team, Dad's crew.

And I managed the next day in school without undue hardship.

After the chickens were gone, we climbed on the shelters for fun.

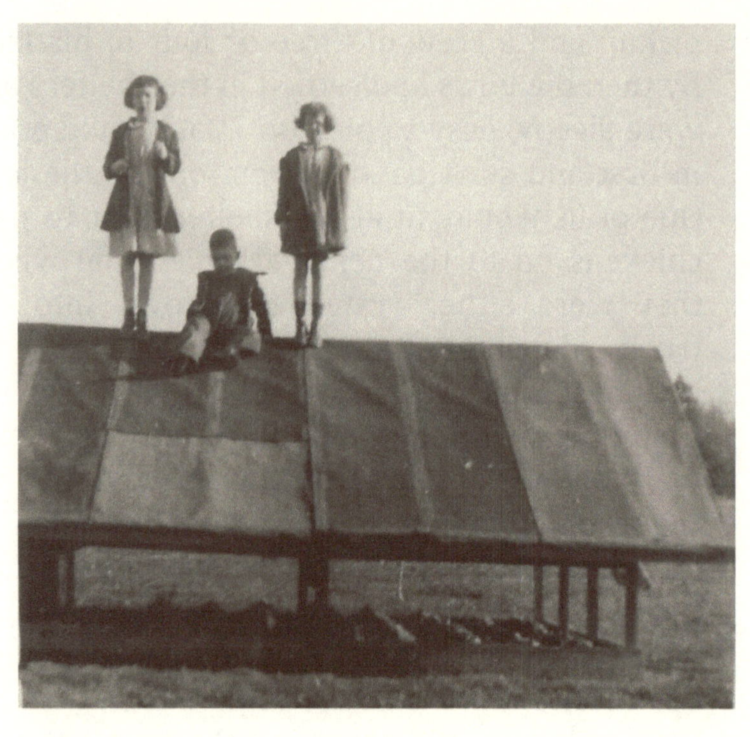

2017. I have added to the handle bars of my exer-bike an elastic sports cord for working my shoulders while I pedal. Ten minutes before breakfast for the legs and shoulders is not a lot but it gets my juices flowing. Later I'll be out walking, a great pleasure and a good way to remind myself about the wide world around. I will stretch and, some days, do a yoga routine.

Food and Exercise among Farmers. Dad lived to 99. Mom was 90 when she died. They worked hard, hiked mountain trails, and gave no thought to exercise. They grew an organic garden before the word organic came into the culture and certainly before organic meant big.

Our first refrigerator was new in 1947. Before that we used an ice box. Dad cut ice every winter, kept it in sawdust in a bin on the shadow side of the barn. The foods we ate from the farm included dairy, chicken, eggs, meat and vegetables, also apples and berries. I remember with delight our trips into the woods to find raspberries or blueberries. Fruits and vegetables were canned in beautiful glass jars.

To make a cake we needed only a dry Betty Crocker mix and eggs and water. Our electric mixer bowl was ingeniously placed on a grooved plate with the beaters off-center to make the bowl turn as they slowly stirred the ingredients.   For biscuits we often used Bisquick, a prepared mix of flour, shortening, and baking powder to which we added water. Not always. We made biscuits from scratch. I learned how to cut shortening into flour for pie crust. Mom had a large board built in under the counter for rolling the crusts. When we were short on butter, Mom bought white margarine with little packets of color we smoothed in.

Once a month, the Cushman came to the house with baked goods. I never knew his name. Mom would buy a jelly roll and a dozen cupcakes, sometimes cream rolls. I can still taste these whipped cream treats with flaky, buttery crusts. There was little danger any of us would eat too many. A dozen didn't go very far in a family of nine. On one occasion, when Mom had seven children ranging from age ten to a few months, she heard my four-year-old brother explain to the Cushman, "Our mother is thirty. Why, she's almost an old maid."

Thoughts of nutrition and exercise were some years away. We ate our meals and we worked and we played. My parents seemed to be no worse for eating processed flour, sugar, and salt, perhaps because their sturdy farming bodies were already in good form. Children are a different case, though. I noticed early on that my youngest sister and I, bottle fed in infancy, were the two who later had trouble with weight gain. We had five siblings who got a better start breastfeeding and did not get the corn syrup until they were several months old. All five have remained slim.

In 1956 the Four Food Groups began to be taught in school and mentioned in magazines. These were 1) dairy, 2) meat, 3) fruits and vegetables, and 4) grains, listed as bread and cereal. No one told us that the meat and dairy industries had promoted the Four Food Groups to induce families to buy their products.

There had been other food guidelines earlier, but those seemed to lack the bias introduced with the Four. Later these were changed to The Food Pyramid and, more recently to The Food Plate. Meanwhile, diet advice seemed to come from every corner. What was an eater to think?

The Family Farm: When Food Became Big Business, 1930 to 1960. In childhood I witnessed another point of view on the food habits of Americans, though understanding came later. Using my father's farm diaries and my memories, I have been able to see the transition from diverse to one crop farming – and then to no farm at all.

My father took over the farm at the age of fifteen when his elderly father became too ill to do the bulk of the work. Dad went to Farm Bureau meetings and discussed farming with Charlie, a young man with the mission of helping area farmers transition to mono-crops. Charlie suggested building a hen house, buying several hundred baby chicks, and selling eggs to a hatchery that would then provide chicks for broiler operations, a direction that would, a few years later, lead Dad to sell his beloved hill farm and move to one where roads were plowed year round. On the hill farm, Dad's uncle and hired help joined the effort and soon there was the first hen house, two floors of pens full of chickens, with a three story addition later.

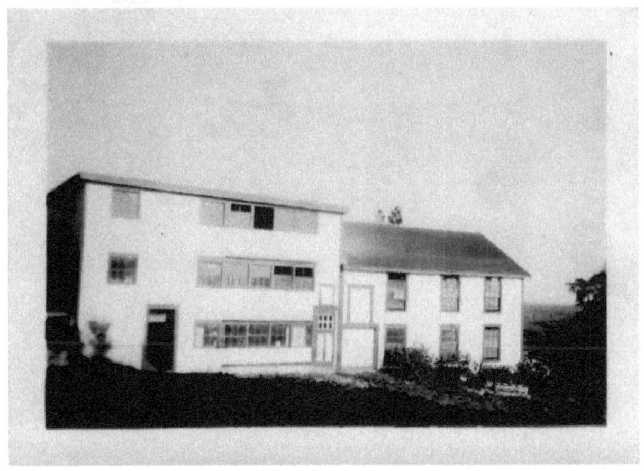

The baby chicks now came not from a mother hen in the barn but by mail in boxes of a hundred. These boxes might spend a night in our living room before Daddy could put them out under the brooders.

There is a story that when I was still a baby in a crib, Daddy came into the living room and found the top off one of the boxes. When he took my toddler sister to task, she pointed to me. "Swishy, Swishy." She had been showing Trishy the chicks. An alternate version of the story says Winky was accusing me of taking the lid off, but Daddy didn't believe that. She was sharing.

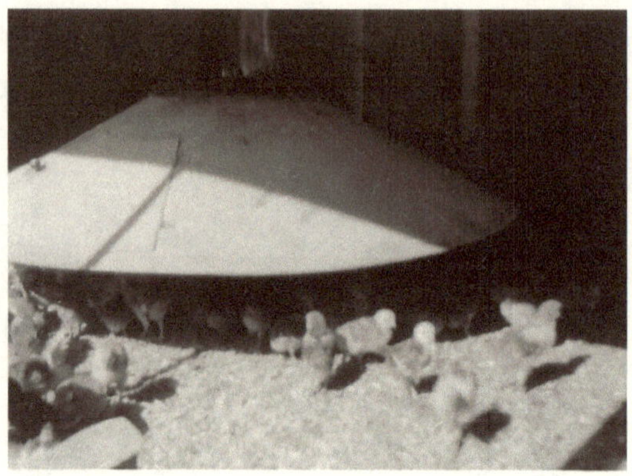

When I was older I liked to put my finger in through one of the air holes to let the newly hatched chicks peck at it.

Dad turned some of the land that had been used for growing market vegetables into a summer range for the chickens. He fenced the range with chicken wire, built rain shelters, and ran water pipes from the windmill.

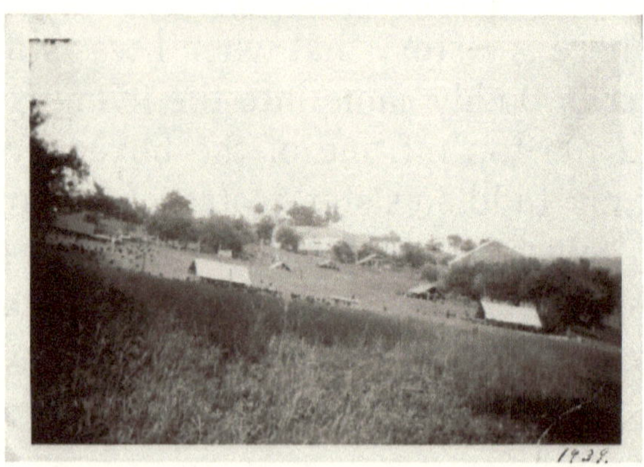

From his childhood on a diversified farm that sold directly to restaurants and homes, Dad had become part of industry. From then on he would continue to keep a couple of cows and a few sheep and to grow a vegetable garden for the family. But the farm's income would come from selling eggs to a hatchery in Delaware. His first flock paid several years of back taxes, making his father proud.

In the beginning Dad was able to make money every year, but after a while he found he lost money every third year. He could manage that and recover. He enjoyed his work and could often be located by listening as he sang opera to the chickens, *The Gypsy Baron, La Traviata, Faust.* When he wasn't singing he was telling tall tales to little daughters as they followed him around. He loved to joke and make us laugh.

There was a cycle: high prices inspired other farmers to raise chickens and sell eggs. The next year the surfeit of eggs brought the prices down. To keep up, Dad built a second henhouse and doubled his output. After a few more years he found he was losing money every other year. To stay solvent he built a grain mill and a couple of silos, ordered wheat, corn, and soy from the Midwest, and ground his own mash. He hired a trucker with a dump truck to haul the beans and grain up the ridge from the train station and dump it in a dumping pit from which it was augured into the silos. From the silos it was ground and mixed in the mill and augured up to the top of the hen house where Dad had built a huge wooden storage bin. From this he opened a chute and carried buckets of mash to a round motorized metal bin attached to feeding trays in which chains moved mash from the front pen through one or two more pens and back around to pick up more grain. It was all amazing to a child.

By then my father was one of only four independent poultry farmers in the state of Maine. As president of the Maine Poultry Association he did his best to encourage independent farmers, and he had no use for the conglomerates that were taking over. I think he read the end of his story in their rise. To counter the pressure from that source, he put flocks of chickens on a couple more farms and hired families to tend them. He sent mash from his mill to the other farms. But Mom noticed that he had in his head so many figures on the price of grain that he had stopped joking. The farms worried him. Like Alice in Lewis Carroll's *Through the Looking Glass,* Dad had to run just to stay in place.

Nor did this narrowing down to chickens appeal to my brother. Any of us children might have been interested in a diversified farm where hens raised their own chicks as they had on the Oak Hill farm, but not in this giant business that our innocent father had created to help his family survive. Had Charlie and the Farm Bureau led Dad astray? Mono-cropping was an economic plan that worked for one generation, just long enough for my father to get his family grown but not long enough to give even one of us a heritage like the Oak Hill farm.

Dad sold the farm, trained in a different skill, and worked for many years for a nearby town, inspecting buildings for code compliance, assessing taxes, and talking calmly with people who were upset about their taxes. Confronted with an angry resident, he would say in his Maine drawl, "Come on into my office. I'll show you how I got those figures." After that the man may still not have liked his tax bill, but he knew it was fair.

By the time it was over, our family had traded our birthright of land for a bowl of food. The Biblical story of Esau and Jacob must have been meant to explain the history of agriculture and the failure that is built into that seemingly wonderful effort. A tribal family that began growing crops could now grow its population beyond what the tribal lands could support and could store food against famine, thus creating the need for walls to keep out hungry others and setting in motion centuries of migration and war.

There's nothing wrong with agriculture. But farming without population control and land husbandry, farming without communication and ethics, can lead only to trouble without end. Furthermore, when two tribes exist side by side, the one with ethics will always lose to the one without. Ask the Six Nations, whose elders wrote *A Basic Call to Consciousness,* what happened to their centuries old successful and graceful culture when the Europeans came.

That's the broad view of what my family experienced. Not that Dad had much choice. We were caught up in the heartache of many farm families. By the twentieth century the transition from multiple crops to one crop was happening all over. And soon enough family farms were mostly gone. It was a trend bad for farmers and bad for our tummies. The new agribusinesses went toward processed food.

I recently read Michael Pollen's terrifying account of how corn was shifted from food to commodity, from farm control to industrial control. In *The Omnivore's Dilemma: A Natural History of Four Meals* (Penguin, 2006), Pollen has this to say:

> What's involved in absorbing all this excess biomass [piles of leftover corn outside granaries in the American

Midwest] goes a long way toward explaining several seemingly unconnected phenomena, from the rise of factory farms and the industrialization of our food to the epidemic of obesity and the epidemic of food poisoning in America, to the fact that in the country where *Zea Mays* was originally domesticated, *campesinos* descended from those domesticators are losing their farms because imported corn, flooding in from the North, has become too cheap. Such is the protean, paradoxical nature of the corn in the pile that getting rid of it could contribute to obesity and hunger both. (page 62)

How's that again? By sending corn to starving people we destroy the farms around those villages and make matters worse? Yikes!

In the United States today some young farmers are returning to small farm production and diversity, giving us the option of avoiding industry meat, processed food, chemical fertilizers, insecticides, and foods that travel thousands of miles to our tables. The big guys are fighting these brave farmers, trying to get laws passed to squeeze them out, increasing the risk of famine.

Famine can make tummies hurt.

If you want to eat in the future, support anyone near you who grows and markets food.

Chefs who start *local food* restaurants with a simple and wholesome menu will be heroes.

When good farmland is sold to developers as was the farm where I grew up, it will never be returned to farming. The good soil will be lost. The good acres will become asphalt and concrete. These are not edible. A group of farmers in Washington County, NY, have agreed not to sell their farms, or to sell only to others who will farm or allow the land to lie fallow in readiness for farming. We need many such groups.

One useful connection came out of my reading of Pollen's chapter on corn. Corn Syrup such as Karo Syrup, and now High Fructose Corn Syrup are taking our health. Bodies need glucose, but a steady diet of glucose interrupts normal metabolism by preventing the storage and release of food. It was something to ponder.

For further reference a bibliography is provided at the end of the book.

2017. Have you heard of an umwich? *You take two or three flat lettuce leaves, add some mayo, sliced turkey, a slice of your favorite cheese, a slice of tomato. Fold your yummy "sandwich" or add another leaf of lettuce and take a bite. I learned this trick because bread, even gluten-free bread, gave me a tummy ache. Then I discovered others doing the same thing. I got the name* umwich *from one of them.*

A Life Begins, 1959. My seventeenth birthday has come and gone. On this late summer evening I am abed. I begin with my usual ritual of expecting to die and wondering if death comes all of a sudden or if there is a warning. Will it hurt? Is there something beyond death or just nothing? I try to imagine nothing, no existence, no awareness, no memory of ever having lived.

I have not told Mom. She would be appalled to learn that her fussing and worrying has translated for me into a belief that I will not live to grow up. Not much sense telling her. She has already done everything she can think of to help me live.

But this evening is different. Lying in my comfortable bed, I think, I'm practically grown now. I've made it. And from now on I will live.
I stopped worrying about dying.

Hiking, 1963. When we could leave the farm in charge of the hired man for a few days, we went camping and hiking. Roaring Brook camp at the base of Mt. Katahdin was a lovely wooded spot equipped with lean-tos, fire rings, and outhouses. Before I returned to college the summer I turned 21, Dad brought several of his children to camp there. We rolled out of our sleeping bags, stowed them in the lean-to, and fixed bacon, eggs, and toast over the campfire, reminding ourselves of what Mom always said: Cooking isn't work if you can do it outdoors.

The trail to Chimney Pond started out as a wide gravel and grass path through the woods. Gradually boulders appeared, at first a few we could walk around. Soon we had to walk on and between boulders, cross ledges, and generally step like goats, a skill learned from many outings in the mountains and along Maine's rocky coastline. We took breaks at the Basin Ponds and at Chimney Pond Campground, admiring the jagged skyline. The sun sparkled on the water, which was clear and tasty. We filled canteens for the last part of the hike, choosing the Cathedral Trail, which meant climbing hand over foot part of the time. At last we reached the plateau and began the less strenuous walk to the peak.

A man and his son who had joined us on the Cathedral Trail were with us when we reached the tall cairn that marks the peak. Many years later I met a man whose uncle had helped build that cairn in the 1930s. The crew carried mix and water to the top, piled up rocks, and secured them with concrete, giving the mountain those last few feet needed to reach the mile high mark. Here is a picture of Mom by the cairn on her honeymoon.

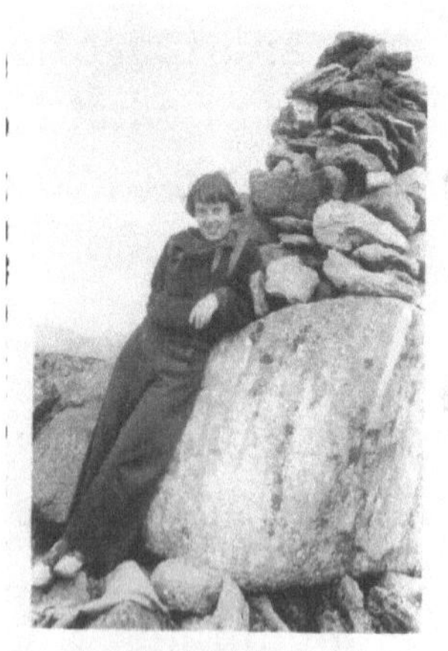

On this later occasion, the man looked around and noticed a three-walled rock fort nearby. "Why do you suppose that structure is there?"

My father explained that it was a fortification left over from Civil War days. Dad went on about the war and the need for defense in the north. He kept a straight face but I was trying not to laugh. The man looked at my face and knew he was listening to a Maine yarn. He laughed. I thought about the many times we children had checked Mom's face to know whether to believe Dad.

Of course Dad leveled with him then. "I expect people built those walls so they could get out of the wind."

With our tummies full of sandwiches and apples, we walked across the plateau and started down the North Basin Trail, a slightly longer and gentler path back to Chimney Pond. I was glad to be going downhill. After awhile we came to place where the trail branched. My brother and sisters went down the other trail a few yards to get a better view. Dad and I stood on at the top, too tired to take extra steps. We had lost our umpf. He was almost fifty and perhaps had an excuse. But what was I doing flagging like that when I should have been in the bloom of youth? I could breathe deeply. My lungs were good. But some invisible ceiling stopped me.

Pictured here are Wayne, Winky, and Dad at the edge of the plateau ready to head down into North Basin.

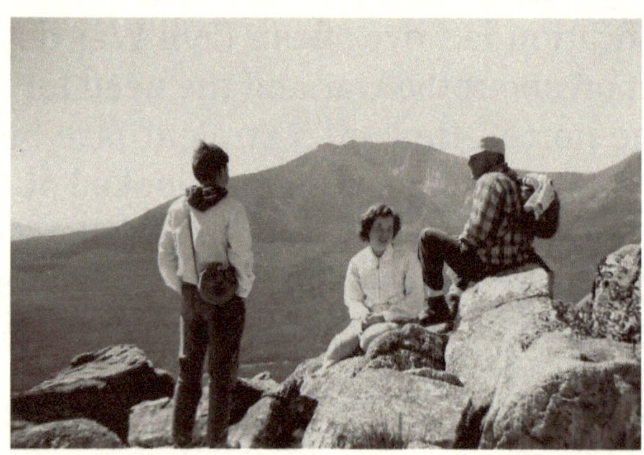

Through the Basin, we hopped along over boulders to Blueberry Knoll where we had the good luck to find ripe berries. From there on down to Chimney Pond and Roaring Brook I was fine. Stepping down was hard on the knees but easy on the umpf.

2017. Living in an apartment on my own is lovely, but it was not my plan. I always meant to end my days in community or extended family, a hands-on grandmother with "sisters" to chat with in the kitchen and gardens.

The Farm in Tennessee and the Farm in the Catskills, 1975 to 1984. We found another farm, until we lost that one as well. In 1975 my husband found on a newsstand a magazine-sized book about The Farm, a community of spiritual hippies in Tennessee. The book was called "Hey Beatnik" and is no longer in print. But you can find The Farm Community on the net. Within a year of moving there my awareness of people and how we arrange ourselves had sharpened and I had begun to understand the threat of multinational corporations bigger than any government and possessed of no allegiance to the people. My medical problems would remain mysterious for some years. But rubbing up against others led me to a strengthening self-confidence and better social skills. I was happy to join the "back to the land" movement with its impulse toward sharing. (See my book *Sweet Potato Suppers: A Yankee Woman Finds Salvation in a Hippie Village*)

In 1980 we moved from that community to a sister Farm in the Catskills where by tribal agreement we co-owned 300 acres in a beautiful valley between hills covered with pines and hemlocks and maple trees. After a few years we lost that land—for much the same reason my father had lost his. It was too hard to make the land pay—in business terms. At first the land was used to grow many acres of vegetables, but when that didn't prove economically sound, the farmers were "strongly invited" to join the one crew that did make money, the construction crew. We had a mortgage and that had to be paid. When your land is mortgaged, you don't really own it. The idealists hoped to find ways to meet the mortgage while continuing to farm, but the pragmatists pointed out the difficulties of doing that.

And so the land was sold, leaving those who still lived there to grieve the loss and scramble for a footing back in mainstream culture—and leaving me to wonder what makes keeping a few acres of land for the people so difficult. What I found out was, you can't wait for economically sound. You have to look for survival beyond economics. (For more about the Farm in the Catskills, see my book *The Farm That Tried to Feed the World: Why Local Farms, Sharing Communities, and Transition Neighborhoods Matter to All of Us.)*

Anything material can fall from your grasp, but life's lessons remain, including the many questions that followed me from community to the single-family-working-mom life considered normal in America. I read books and talked to friends about raising kids, about health and lifestyle, all intertwined. During those years several strong books came into my hands. I felt my way among the ideas, cautiously at first and yet willing to believe most anything, provisionally, while I explored.

2017. Before breakfast I cook for the day and set lunch out. Hypoglycemia can come on fast and I don't take chances. One minute fine and the next, every cell screaming collapse. A person suffering from low blood glucose is not going to lie down and look sick. We prowl like hungry tigers. Oddly, when I have eaten my day's fill, my body purrs through the evening and night hours.

1978, The Sun House. In one of the larger houses in our communal village, I wake up early and as cheerful as my smiling baby. I change him and his toddler brother. Together with my six-year-old we go downstairs to breakfast, a meal of coarse wheat cereal served with margarine and sugar. I eat while I nurse the baby. The cereal is yummy. My children empty their bowls. The oldest runs off to play. The toddler joins a friend in rrmming little cars across the floor.

Breakfast is satisfying. But by the time I have folded the laundry someone kindly took from the lines and piled on my bed, my *juice* is gone. Back down in the kitchen I find one of the women frying tofu her boy lugged home from the soy dairy in a bucket. She has biscuits in the oven. No fruit or vegetables available just now. We make do. I'm glad she doesn't need me. The baby needs to nurse again and I'm grateful. I can't stay on my feet another minute. From the couch I watch her truck around the kitchen, her energy never flagging. How does she do it? Is she more dedicated than I? More spiritual? More willing to be in pain and pretend she is not? I'm too weak to stand up without lunch. It would be painful to try. I worry I might faint. This would be clearly a health red flag, but no one in the household trusts me enough to see it, and I don't trust myself.

After lunch I feel good. My juice is back. But I feel drugged and dragged into sleep. I take the babies up to bed and lie down for a snooze, leaving my older child to play with the other household children.

After the twenty minute nap my head is clear and the drugged feeling has lifted. I check on my oldest and sweep the hall and stairs, listening for the babies. I get them up, change diapers, nurse, read stories—and wait desperately for supper. I'm out of energy. Supper comes at last. I put my children to bed and fall asleep nursing the baby. Before sleep takes me I vow tomorrow I will do my share.

I never do my share.

I'm afraid to start anything I will be unable to finish, afraid of the pain of having to keep standing and rolling tortillas for forty people.

Each day the same pattern repeats, a good start, the slump before lunch, lunch at last, the drugged nap, the slump before supper, supper at last, the drugged bedtime.

I am sick. But no one knows that. The other women get mad at me for not doing my share. We have long *sort-outs* about it, talks that make me feel thrown away, a repeat of a childhood pattern.

And let's be clear about illness. Bodies are rugged, built to thrive and do with ease the many tasks we require of them. A body living in an ancestral area and eating good traditional food will run smoothly. But we are many generations out from our ancestral lands on a journey through illness and back to health.

Deep in Trouble, 1983. It is midnight on a summer night in August. I am driving home from second shift at Job Corp, an economic opportunity school for low income youth. Since most students reside on campus, Resident Advisors like me work afternoon and evening hours when the students are not in class. On the drive up Franklin Mountain toward my home in the country, I keep looking at the car clock and wishing the trip faster. If I can be in bed by one o'clock, I'll get five hours of sleep by six when my little boys will be chirping, my husband out the door for work. This was my third week on the job—first job since the youngest child was born. Night rolls by my car windows. Cool air comes in, helping me stay awake. I make a decision. I cannot go on. Even a more robust mother would have found the schedule challenging.   I remember Dick Gregory's story about his beloved mother who worked herself into an early grave for the sake of her children. I'm not ready to settle for an early death. There has to be a better way.

Luck. The next day I learn of a September opening for a Family Counselor at Head Start. With two boys in school and the youngest with me at Head Start, I can manage.

Nutrition. Head Start has been praised for feeding low income children as well as teaching them basic social skills. What child can learn when her tummy is empty? I still recall the delicious mac and cheese served at a typical Head Start lunch. However, for me the diet was ruinous. After a decade of eating home-ground, unprocessed wheat, this was my first taste of bleached and processed flour, processed again into noodles. I began my work there at 112 lbs. By the time I left more than a year later I weighed over 120. I haven't seen 112 since. Nor has my family had the excellent nutrition of my days as a stay-at-home mother. I doubt the program could afford local butter and cheese even though there were dairy farms all around.

The 1980s were the beginning of the age of obesity. The formula goes like this: Poverty leads to hunger leads to cheap food leads to getting fat without getting full leads to hunger.... A greedy food industry was more than happy to provide cheap, empty food.

Fighting for my own health and energy, I was also fighting our tragic descent from food integrity to the travesty of food that looks like food but lacks nutritional value. Go into any supermarket and look at a lovely, large, unblemished yellow pepper. If it's been grown on land from which the nutrients have long been sucked out by former crops or leached away, you don't see an actual pepper, only the form of one. In *The Omnivore's Dilemma* Michael Pollen gives us some of the science showing what happens to food grown in depleted soils. For one thing, plants that don't get to grow their own immune systems don't have the ingredients we need for ours. (page 180)

A *Twilight Zone* episode showed scientists offering a group of people a substance that looks something like a cream-colored sponge. They say, "Eat it and imagine any food you want. It will taste like that food." The people try it and find a banquet of food available. But afterwards, real food tastes to them like sawdust.

We now know that the new "foods" are made out of corn twisted and tweaked in a hundred ways into anything you can imagine. And the people have no taste for real food.

The children I met at Head Start and, later, as caseworker in an outreach program for young mothers, had mostly not been breastfed. After World War II, Medical Doctors were more listened to than the wise women of the family and neighborhood. MDs advised bottle feeding, having somehow been convinced that formula was better for babies than mother's milk. At first it was the well-to-do who took up the latest in infant feeding, but soon the poorest family in the hills found out what high status women were doing, and they wanted it too. Sometimes a baby did get better nutrition from a bottle—if the mother was not healthy and eating well. But formulas lacked the immune support of mother's milk and, as well, the microbes every working tummy needs. Fortunately, most pediatricians today try to reverse that trend. Mother's milk is best. And science is firmly on the side of breast milk. (See Jennifer Verdolin, *Raised by Animals,* page 112)

In the 1980s I was trying to persuade a pregnant teen to consider breastfeeding. I mentioned that it is much cheaper for the nursing mother to eat well than to buy formula. She looked at me with what seemed like a mixture of hurt and stubborn pride. "My baby deserves bottles and formula just like every other baby in this county." One young father-to-be said, "Her breasts are mine and I don't want that baby touching them." Or, how about the girl who put soda in the bottle? She did it partly because soda was cheaper and they didn't always have formula, and also in the spirit of sharing. "Whatever I have, she gets too." What were the chances that her child would grow up to be an intelligent, contributing member of society? More likely, she would spend her life on welfare like her mother.

Home visits like that broke my heart. I'd think, There but for the grace of God go I. I was powerless to stop the descent of our society into the decades of empty eating that have followed. When had life become so complicated and confused that these young parents had no one they were willing to trust, no one who deserved their trust?

The Exhausted Mother, 1998. When I was
raising my children I wanted to take them
places on weekends. There was an animal farm
we never got to. There was our small city to
explore and learn about. But working full time
and caring for the household left me with
nothing to spare. I depended utterly on my
routine, bedtime at 9:30 pm, housecleaning on
Saturday mornings, naps when I could get them
or I'd be beside myself with fog and fatigue by
evening.

When one of our sons was in his teens and
not yet driving, he took a job at a fast food
restaurant, walking to work or getting rides

with friends. But we didn't allow him to walk home after dark. My husband had been providing rides. Then there came a night when Don was working second shift and Ben needed a ride home at eleven. What could I say? Of course I would do it, much though I knew it would cost me dearly to be up so late. I drove over at eleven and parked on the near side where I could clearly see Ben mopping a floor. He seemed leisurely and not a bit concerned that it was eleven. I sat and watched, getting more and more upset. Why was he not ready to leave when he said he would be? By the time he looked up and saw my car it was twenty after eleven and I was steamed. He got in the car.

I let him have it. "Why did you leave me sitting here for twenty minutes? You said eleven."

"I didn't see your car. Don always parks on the other side. I was watching over there."

Oh! What a mix-up. I should have let go of my anger. The confusion and my exhaustion were not Ben's fault. But, I was too wasted to stop arguing. When we got home Don, just getting in himself, settled us down by explaining each of us to the other.

Living on the edge of exhaustion didn't keep me from tending a family and earning a paycheck. I was a thorough and devoted mother, though my illness, which by then I thought was due entirely to yeast overgrowth caused by antibiotics, cost my children. Fortunately they were good boys and more helpful than not. The oldest began to do his own laundry before he was a teenager and the others followed his example.

Where I lacked stamina I substituted heart, giving the children quality attention from birth on. At work I brought to my girls, and to their guys and babies, respect and love, the only theory of social work that matters. I also brought baby furniture, clothing, supplies, and whatever guidance they would accept. It was my good fortune to do what I loved and keep my own calendar, set my own pace. I kept the job for almost twenty years from the time my youngest went to kindergarten until all three were grown. My salary paid for groceries, clothes, shoes, and school fees. It made music lessons possible and gave our family the occasional meal out to celebrate good report cards. It paid for the phone, a black wall phone with a circular dial and long cord. If you can't picture such a phone, you are not alone. There is a lovely moment in Barbara Kingsolver's novel *Flight Behavior* where a toddler is pulling a toy phone around by the speaker piece and the grandmother wants to know why she doesn't speak into it. The mother says, "She doesn't know it's a phone."

I'm sure no one makes toy phones with dials and speakers today. A toy phone would have to look like a cell phone.

2017. I have found an herbal treatment for UTIs, a pesky problem that would otherwise send me to urgent care for ciprofloxacin, an antibiotic. I hope to continue finding alternatives. I have had all the antibiotics my tummy can handle.

Antibiotics, 1948 to 2017. Penicillin at age six was the only antibiotic I took until my early thirties when I had bronchitis, which, if I remember correctly, was treated with tetracycline. After that there was another long gap when I had only the occasional cold, with no call for a trip to the doctor. Then, when I was almost sixty, I had a series of seeming colds and a sinus infection discovered when I went to the dentist, who prescribed augmentin to resolve the infection before he could give me two root canals.

Yikes!

Hard on the tummy.

I'm not saying we'd have been better off to go back to the early 1900s before antibiotics were available. Those were not the good old days. Civilization had already slipped from the natural health we once knew. Disease and plague came along with over-population and crowding. Antibiotics seemed a miracle because we needed a miracle—or a few million.

My next dose of antibiotics was five years later, doxycycline for a tick infection. At almost seventy, I was twice prescribed ciprofloxacin for UTIs. That same summer I had another tick bite and another round of doxy. Concurrently, and for a couple of years, I had a sinus infection that finally could only be resolved with surgery, after which the doctor gave me amoxicillin to prevent infection.

My tummy rebelled. One week of amoxicillin upset my system so thoroughly I couldn't eat or sleep. After walking the floor all night to get the gas up, I went to the ER exhausted and dehydrated. I assumed the culprit was yeast. Perhaps it had been hiding and was now back on the rampage, what with three rounds of antibiotics in one year.

Couple months later, more cipro for another UTI. Ouch! This was getting scary. How much could a beleaguered tummy take?

It was at about that time I met Dr. Jenkins, a local Alternative Medicine doctor who generously took time during Chiropractic visits to talk with me about general health concerns. Finding him was a turning point.

But even with support from alternative medical models I was not able to avoid taking yet more antibiotics in the spring of 2017. Here is an abridged version of an entry I made on facebook one bleak evening when I unknowingly had a throat infection and pneumonia, complaints that would take me to urgent care in the morning. The title I have the entry was, "Someone to Watch over Me: Why Old People Complain about their Health."

You would think we would be eager to avoid becoming that cliché of an old person who talks and talks, in detail, about their ill health. One man went to a class reunion and reported back to his wife that it was more of an organ recital.

We get it. We've been to those reunions. Many of us have added ours to the chant of body troubles. And if by chance we are stoic enough not to join in, it's not because we don't have anything to contribute. "Old age is not for sissies." No doubt the adage goes back centuries. The little aches and pains we were able to ignore when we were younger have grown bigger and piled up. We are dealing now with indigestion and a sinus headache and a lame toe all at once, and the things we do to settle these troubles don't work as well as they used to.

I had an uncle who was the lead singer in a band. One song's chorus went, "Some little bug'll get you someday." The verses were each dedicated to a particular illness.

What is behind the urge to complain—and also laugh—about our health?

It's late at night. I'm alone. My throat hurts and I'm all stuffed up and how can I sleep if I can't breathe. Help! I want my mommy.

As children, all we had to do was tell our mother and she would go into action—wash a scraped knee and put a Band-aid on it, take our temperature, give us cough syrup. If you were lucky you had a mommy like that or maybe a daddy or a grampa or that special aunt who always arrived when you were sick and mom had to go to work.

You are a fortunate elder if you have a spouse willing to listen and feel your forehead, someone who is there to drive you to the doctor if needed. But not every spouse is attentive and many elders don't have a partner. We are alone with our ills. I like living alone when I'm feeling well, but when I'm bad sick I want my mommy.

Part of the trouble is in our housing and social arrangements. Throughout history people have lived in tribes or in villages and neighborhoods, often next door to a sister or other near relative. But I live in an apartment building where I have the dubious luxury of my own space where I can be self-sufficient and where I could presumably be sick and even die without anyone knowing for days. Of course, we check on those we haven't seen lately. And, because it is senior housing, we have pull-cords in our bedrooms and bathrooms.

But why should it be an emergency before we have someone to help us when we are ill? Why not a sister who cooks over the same fire or a daughter who checks on us easily because we live in an extended family household? More, what has happened to that shared body of knowledge about how to stay well or regain health? Where are the healers and remedies of yesteryear?

That built-in village is what we are looking for when we mention our health concerns. Each body breakdown, whether small or large, reminds us of our mortality. And most don't want to die alone.

As for me, the only thing to do is brave up. Some little bug or body breakdown will get each of us someday. And we may well be alone. Heck, if it's a sudden illness or accident, we may not even be at home. A friend was at church one evening where the message was, "The Devil's Gonna Get You." If that wasn't warning enough, during her trip home that foggy evening her car radio caught another sermon admonishing, "The Devil's Gonna Get You." White-knuckled on the steering wheel, she prayed, "Let the Devil not get me until I get home."

Okay, if I'm going to talk about being brave then I have to face my own death. Don't get me wrong. I'm willing to die. Just not yet. I have grandchildren to love and friends to cherish and stories to write. I'm too busy to die.

I'll stop expecting my friends and family to be my mommy. At the same time, I will listen to the complaints of others in a deeper way. They only want what we all want, someone to watch over us.

2017. If I get up at seven I must eat by eight, a full meal, usually an egg steamed with broccoli, carrots, and kale or some other mix of vegetables. I put butter on my egg because I have learned that my body runs best on fat. For one, the adrenals make hormones out of cholesterol. I looked it up.

We the People, 1776 and 2017. First take a look around at the health of the people. Americans are sick. We expect to die of heart attacks and strokes, diabetes and cancer, and we keep doing it in large numbers. No matter what we've been told about how to prevent those terrible diseases, we can't seem to improve our statistics. We don't know what we are doing wrong. Most of us have lost all connection with the wisdom that comes of knowing a land and its ways, and that includes knowing what to eat. Most of us came here from other lands. Even if our ancestors came on the Mayflower, as some of mine did, we are still immigrants. We have been uprooted again and again as violence swept across our first villages and then across our adopted lands. We don't know what to eat and what not to eat. To judge by the use of doctors and hospital emergency rooms we don't know how to treat even minor illnesses at home.

Who are we? What have we become?

When our founders began *The Constitution of the United States* with "We the people," they could not have imagined what we would become in a couple of centuries. In their day "the people" were educated and aware. The grade schools Jefferson urged the new nation to provide turned out graduates who knew more than most college graduates today. They learned in school and they learned from the people around them just as children today learn to handle smart phones at a young age. The delegates who signed the document were also farmers. Everyone kept horses and grew food. A few ran small businesses in town: a bakery, a hardware store, a butcher shop. Clothes were mostly made at home from cloth woven at home. These were able people. There was no welfare or Social Security until the 1930s. Your security was your network of neighbors and family. You made a contribution to the survival of the village, and you received help when you were down. A man who broke a leg falling off a horse knew that neighbors would show up to feed and milk his cows.

Every village had a midwife or two—and every woman was a midwife, knowing how to boil water and coax a baby into the world, when the need arose. You'll say that many mothers and babies died. True. Already health was degenerating. Women were losing trust in their own bodies and holding themselves against the process of birth. Childbed fever had become a big concern. The Europeans who settled this continent were a sick people compared to those indigenous to the land. Not that I learned any of this in school. I learned it by reading alternate history.

Even with the diseases they brought here from Europe, the people were mostly sturdy and self-sufficient. They were survivors. Somehow I don't think Jefferson would expect the people we have become to survive.

Gut, 2017. The condition of the gut is said to be at the base of good health. With its bacterial and yeastly residents and its job of breaking down and absorbing food, the gut determines the health of the rest of the body, from the condition of the organs, muscles, and systems, to the clarity of the brain. The digestive tract is a pink tube that runs through the middle of the body yet is outside the body. It readies food for use and guides the transfer from out to in.

Health detective work used to be hard for the lay person, owner of just one body. Mysteries were common. Thankfully, by the time I started my spa, resources were more readily available. It still took persistence.

Gathering information about the connection between the gut and the rest of the body has been like living an ancient fairy tale where it was necessary to find helpers and keys. Helpers were scarce in the early years, abundant now. Sometimes a key found in one decade of life finally fit a door in another. For example, my left arm used to ache, and that can be a sign of a distressed heart. But my EKG's were normal. It wasn't until the past year that I connected that symptom with low potassium. Now an achy left arm reminds me to take more potassium—and to eat my fruits and veggies. The journey has required emotional umpf when physical umpf was in short supply.

The journey has paid off.

I know now why my tummy hurts and, possibly, why yours hurts. If you are among those who received an antibiotic such as penicillin in childhood, and if you got a lot of it, the natural mix of beneficial gut bacteria and yeast were mostly wiped out. Your digestion has perhaps never worked as it was meant to work.

Without modern surgery and antibiotics, my parents would have raised only four of their seven children. How can we not be grateful? Penicillin saved my life. But it was a fumbling sort of save that brought with it hidden complications—most importantly, wrong yeasts and wrong bacteria. These bad guys happily grew fat on the wrong food I ate, including processed flour and sugar. The bad bugs were invisible and never came to the minds of doctor or parents. But they gave me and all of us a bewildering array of troubles. According to Michael Pollen, processing twists into ever new contortions. Where once there was Karo Syrup, we now have High Fructose Corn Syrup, and this dangerous processed corn is in much of what you can buy in the central isles of your store. Then there are chemicals added to improve color or lengthen shelf life. If I start to read the label on a product and see a long list of ingredients I put it back. Simple food is more likely to be real food.

Our tummy aches and all complaints linked to digestion are something we as a people have needed to go through—worth it if we find out what caused the trouble and make changes. The arc of any good story is from innocence to wisdom.

2017. This year my daughter-in-law showed me how to make no grain brownies that are nutritious and delicious. I'm lucky to have her to consult and imitate. She is a chef of tasty meals and a busy mama who wants the best for her family. The grandkids are thriving. Oh, and she feeds my son well. At forty he is slim and healthy.

Feeding a Family in the 90s. I didn't know whether I could get my health back but I was grateful to be able to get the next generation started off well. My babies were wanted and planned for. I ate well while I was pregnant. I birthed the first by Lamaze at Boston Lying In where I loved my doctors' hands off attitude. They mostly just smiled with me. The second and third were born at home in the care of trained spiritual midwives. The word *spiritual* meant that they were kind and respectful to the laboring mother and the new child, regarding both as spiritual beings. My babies were breastfed. All three were slim and healthy throughout childhood. Ours was not a junk food house, partly because I was not eating sugars or processed snacks.

Our favorite family meals were homemade tortillas and pinto beans with all the fixings; chicken soup; and tofu spaghetti with oven-warmed garlic bread. When we needed a faster supper, I served toasted English muffins made into little pizzas. Doing my best to keep our diet healthy, I served vegetables with all meals—which the kids mostly ate without complaint.

Still, they were normal children. During one meal the youngest listened politely to my lecture that green beans were full of vitamins and minerals. He said, "Well, what shall we do, pray my tongue changes?"

2017. Our building is set in the woods and has a walkway around it. This morning I walked with a friend and talked about making a quiche with a sweet potato bottom instead of a wheat crust. We talked about our families and were happy together.

Hiking East Rock, 2009. Several years ago a friend and I decided to walk one of the trails up East Rock, a cliff that rises in the city of New Haven parallel to West Rock, with which I was familiar. We didn't know the East Rock trails.

We started up a promising path and followed it a ways. But it petered out. By then we had invested enough time that we didn't want to turn back. East Rock is not very big, we thought. We decided to cut across a small ridge at a slant and meet up with a trail beyond. She went ahead and managed a steep section, then planted herself behind a tree to offer me a hand. When I crawled and pulled up to her, I found we had another steep knoll to master. The further we went the less we wanted to give up. Surely we would reach a trail soon. Over one more ridge we found the trail and made our way toward it on a downward slant.

By then I was shaking, able only to get back to where we had parked the car. I continued to shake. Desperate for energy, I chewed a sandwich. I could not account for my extreme exhaustion. We were not climbing Mt. Everest, nor even Mt. Katahdin. What was the matter with me?

I was not to find out until 2017 while I was writing this book. It was not hypoglycemia, though that disorder of the pancreas also plagued me more as I grew older.

2017. Reading and living. Apparently hypoglycemia, or low blood glucose, comes from an imbalance of the hormones needed to store and use the food we don't burn right away. I'm no expert, but I know what I experience and I know when my body's ways correspond with what the books say. An imbalance would come from a disruption of the making of those hormones.

Hypoglycemia, 1942 to 2017. A body's inability to regulate glucose levels in the bloodstream is a most unwelcome problem. In my personal health spa, if Tricia the provider didn't keep healthy meals coming, Tricia the patient would be forced to grab anything she could find, making problems for both tummy and metabolism. Confession: when I'm writing I tend to neglect my duties. I ask myself what's the sense in tending a body to the exclusion of living? Well, hypoglycemia makes me pay.

I quit one doctor after trying in vain to describe the way hypoglycemia feels. After listening without listening, he said, "So, I guess you are just really hungry, right?" No, Doctor.

Sometimes I don't even want to eat. My tummy begs for a long vacation, a good fast. But every cell in my body is crying *help!* My brain, my muscles, my organs, my blood all say, "Feed us or we will shut down." It is terrifying. When my blood glucose begins to sink with no food available, I panic. I get agitated. This show of energy convinces others that I can't be too bad off or I'd act sick.

One Physician's Assistant in an ER saw my frantic state and started asking me about my mental health. Meanwhile, they brought me a can of ginger ale, which I drank with huge relief even knowing that I had just swallowed HFCS, or High Fructose Corn Syrup, which is Karo squared. It worked. Suddenly I didn't need to be in the ER. I had been dangerously low on glucose even after breakfast that morning, scared enough to go to the ER. But the ER is never the answer for this condition. After that I learned to carry glucose tabs. And to stock just one sugary soda for emergencies. By long habit, I carry food with me everywhere.

This part of my story hooks in with the plight of small farmers, those near us and many around the world. While processed grains, especially corn, continue to flood the markets, and while we continue to buy these questionable products, we are undermining our future food supply and that of our grandchildren.

The human body was built to withstand limited times of starvation. In *The Old Way*, Elizabeth Marshall Thomas describes three-day hunting forays during which, in order to be fleet of foot, hunters of the Kalahari take no food and little water. They shoot an antelope and then run after it for a day or more until it drops. There they roast a portion of the kill and feast before shouldering the rest to bring back to the people. (*The Old Way: A Story of the First People*, 2006)

Such endurance would not have been possible for me any time in this life. Like many hypoglycemics, I am as vulnerable to starvation as the newborn baby I was when my mother put corn syrup in my milk. I suppose a dose of glucose every few hours must have prevented my pancreas from producing glucagon, the hormone opposite insulin. My body never learned to burn fat, necessary for a strong metabolism. The cow's milk she gave me didn't have much fat in it. The cream was skimmed off to make butter. Still, the milk she gave me did have a value she could not have known.

But I'm getting ahead of myself. I only just found out one special value of that early version of baby formula.

2017. Winter skin. My apartment will absorb a couple of gallons of water every twenty-four hours and still be dry enough to cause my thin skin to itch to the point of pain. I check the warm mist humidifier for water and also add water to an open crock pot I keep going. In the middle of the day I open windows, turn on exhaust fans. I want fresh air, oxygen, moisture. I try various lotions, anti-itch creams and healing balms.

The Insults of Aging, 1980 to 2017. My three chronic conditions, hypoglycemia, an unhappy tummy, and low stamina, didn't exempt me from other insults of aging. Of course, everyone ages differently and at different rates. I like to be careful what I put down to *aging.*

There was a man who consulted a doctor because his leg hurt. The doctor said it was just age. The man said, "That can't be. After all, my other leg is the same age and it doesn't hurt."

Dismissing a problem as due to age could prevent one from looking for the cause. Still, there are some things that do seem to belong to the slow progression of aging. I remember the first time my butt muscles failed to cover my bones the way they had for forty some years. I drew some bath water, got in, sat down—and felt the muscles slide off and allow the sitz bones to thunk on the tub enamel. What was that all about? It seemed uncalled for and suggested other thunks to come.

Or, sometimes a whisper. When I was over fifty, I began to have an occasional odd fluttery feeling in the top of my chest. Not a big concern but it made me feel vaguely unwell. I'd ask my doctors about it. I'd say, "It's just a flutter here. Almost not a physical feeling." None of my doctors in twenty years had a clue. Was this "just aging?"

My uncle once told the story of sitting with a friend in a bar and seeing, across the way, the back of a man's head. He pitied the man because he had developed a bald spot. Then my uncle realized there were two mirrors involved and he was seeing the back of his own head. I thought of my uncle when my glorious long hair began to thin and pull out because of its weight. If I wanted to keep any hair I had to cut it. Now I look in the mirror and wonder who that is. I laugh at myself for the years of believing that younger look was me. This is a body I'm fond of but it is temporary. It is not me.

A couple years ago my grandson, age three, ran his finger over the back of my hand. "Grammie, why do your hands look like that?" I told him they were old hands. I said, "These hands are seventy-two years old." We admired his smooth young hands. The next morning at breakfast he asked, "Grammie, do you still have *old hands*?" I held them up for him to inspect. Children are scientists. Did old hands in the evening mean old hands next morning?

Then came the itching and sneezing. I had never had allergies. Now I was reacting to pollens, molds, and dust. I felt abused. Why me? But I could not get stuck in self pity. I put allergies on my list of mysteries and began watching for clues. If I was not a health professional, I was a professional user of one body and I had a good memory for all I had been through. I had a feeling that everything tied together somehow even if I didn't yet see the lines of connection.

For most people, aging can be slowed down with good diet and exercise. For an upbeat view, please see *Younger Next Year* by Chris Crowley and Henry S. Lodge, M.D. (Workman Publishing, NY, 2004, 2007). They take a *can do* approach and use exercise to mimic our ancient activities of hunting and gathering.

2017. My dream of raising children without parent inflicted trauma has now reached the next generation. My sons are tender fathers. They married good women who really like them. Meanwhile, I've published a number of books (books are my other children), each out of a passion for sharing insights that come from error and pain—and from winning through.

A Healing Trend. Let's swing back up to sane and simple, to the medical traditions and knowledge that have emerged—or re-emerged—in recent years, and to the best that medical science can do in partnership with these older ways.

Diagnosis is fun. Here is a family story about diagnoses—and the fun of solving problems. When the plumbing in a house we had recently bought proved inadequate for a family of five, we called a plumber. He couldn't figure the problem out, so we called the Roto-Rooter. The Roto-Rooter man ran a metal snake down the drain to where it bumped up against concrete. He said, "You'll have to get a backhoe and dig up the lawn."

My husband walked around wringing his hands at the thought of what that would cost. But his friend Scotty said, "Oh boy, oh boy, we're gonna get that backhoe over here and then we'll see some action." I let the boys stay home from school to watch. The backhoe dug down to a cistern. The old lady who had lived in that house for many years had somehow avoided the mandate to hook up to the town sewer line. We figure she must have bribed someone.

Regarding attitude, I was glad the boys had Scotty's example to compare with their father's. Of course, Scotty wasn't paying the bill. Yet, somehow it seems best to meet life's challenges with relish.

At about the time I went to work for Head Start and found that a full day of work and another of house and children took more stamina than I had, I learned of an MD who was into alternative medicine. She was the first to mention Candida as a diagnosis. She gave me Nystatin, a weak medication that only helps if you don't eat sugar. It made work and family possible.

A few years later another MD, a caring man, repeated the diagnosis and continued the Nystatin. Then, the German healer Hannah Kroeger was able to spot my problem as Candida from a saliva sample I sent, dried, on a paper towel. For years I took the Kantita capsules her company prepared. The capsules made my busy life almost okay. Composed of an herbal formula, they reduced the yeast in my system enough to spare me many symptoms, including headaches, weariness, stomach distress, and feeling crappy all over. My evening prayer was, Lord, Please keep me alive until my children are grown.

Hannah Kroeger, heir to an ancient European tradition, has helped many people connect back to traditional medicine, long forgotten in our allopathic world. I read her books and found them useful.

By the time my boys were off to college, I hit a low of a different kind. Something was going badly out of balance. For some four years I depended on a Chinese Medicine practitioner to test my pulses and supply me with supporting herbs to boil and drink. She helped steady a deteriorating system—but she could not heal me. I had had heart palpitations for some years and these were getting worse. I had taken a medicine called *atenalol* which one doctor said would give me five extra years of life as compared to those who didn't take it. But it lowered my already low blood pressure. Standing in line to buy groceries I often had the feeling I would faint before I could get through the line. I stopped taking *atenalol*. I have almost never taken any chemical medicine

more than very short term. They never seemed
to work for me.

I was a social worker visiting teen parents.
One work day I was driving into the hills on
home visits. I was fifty-nine and sicker than I
had been before. I felt shaky and low. The
herbal tea had helped but I was losing my grip.
I was on a slippery log high over a stream.

Was this the end for me?

I had made it further than I ever expected. I
had enjoyed my life fully, even the hardships.
At the remembered pleasure of little boys at my
side, a deep sigh breezed across my hands on
the steering wheel. Such good friends, my
young children. Such good friends my grown
boys.

My thoughts go like this: What will my
husband and children do without me? I won't
be there to provide that glue we women give a
family or to mediate troubles. The boys are in
their twenties, that wonderful decade when
everything is possible and much not yet
learned. I don't want to leave until I see them
better settled.

Playing on the car tape player is *Horowitz,
The Poet,* a collection in which the great pianist
plays a Robert Schumann piece of such
sweetness and triumph it pierces my heart.

Yes! I want my children to play this piece at
my memorial service. I want them to know I

won. I had lived this long against odds, and I had enjoyed my life.

But wait. A rescue was on the way in the form of Nutrition Response Testing.

2017. Once a month when the weather is mild I get into my 1993 Subaru and travel to southern Massachusetts to have my body's systems checked. When I arrive with time to wait, I watch a video in which Freddie Ulan demonstrates Nutrition Response Testing. This morning he is treating a young man who seems in good health except he has lost upper body strength. Going through a basic routine, Freddie notices on the young man's left upper arm an extensive tattoo. "Here's the problem," he says. The tattoo needle had hit some of the nerve network in the skin. Freddie sends the man to his team behind the scenes for treatment.

Nutrition Response Testing, 2002 to the Present. A chance acquaintance connected me with The Natural Health Improvement Center in Glens Falls, NY, Freddie Ulan's clinic. My heart was doing jumps again and she thought I should consult with Freddie. He put me through some tests and determined that the organ that needed the most support was the thyroid.

I said. "My doctor tests for thyroid problems and tells me mine is fine."

"Those blood tests miss about fifty percent of thyroid problems," he said.

He gave me a whole food supplement to support the thyroid. Within two weeks I felt my energy surge. Freddie's Nutrition Response Testing technique was based on applied kinesiology which tests the strength of muscles in relationship to problems and treatments.

It was under Freddie's guidance I first got in the habit of eating an egg with a mix of broccoli and carrots or kale and sweet potatoes, my usual breakfast now fifteen years later. I had always liked vegetables. I'm astonished when I meet up with people who don't. Still, I know people who don't eat anything like what Freddie advised and who yet, with their metabolism and without the problems I have had, live happily into a fine old age. Changing the diet is for people who are struggling, people who are searching for answers because their own habits and preferences have failed them.

I have had people question the validity of muscle testing, even members of my own family who think I have been deluded—though why anyone would think I'd stay with it if it didn't work, puzzles me. I do understand their doubts, though. In a culture where hidden things go on, it is easy to be suspicious. And if, like me, you have lost trust in the "truths" of your youth, you may take many a dead end path before finding one that guides you though.

NRT may not impress a well person and can even seem a little spooky if you don't know about the electrical field that surrounds the body. But what did I have to lose? I was too sick to quibble. Sometimes help comes to us when we need it most, help we might reject if we weren't backed against a wall. In my case, Nutrition Response Testing has proven itself. My NRT docs have diagnosed and treated any number of ills my regular doctor wasn't finding with his very different protocols. They have found three metal toxicities: mercury in 2005, aluminum in 2009, and nickel in 2012.

Toxicity means poison. Poison blocks healing.

Each of those times I was stuck. I had to detox. I was apparently more susceptible to metal exposures than most. I can suppose it had to do with my long term problems with digestion and the conditions that followed. But that was not the whole story.

Yoga, 1994 to 2017. We in the West have benefitted in recent years by greater contact with Eastern practices than our parents and grandparents had. Yoga postures, for example, were developed through many centuries to enhance the body's strengths and flexibilities. In a comprehensive program of postures, every muscle, bone, and group of connecting tissues gets stretched and strengthened. What a boon to be able to tap into those centuries of wisdom.

I had become a head floating above a stiffening body over which I had little control. Then, when I was over fifty, I discovered yoga. Not that I hadn't heard about yoga most of my adult life, but I had never found out what it was. That's the trouble with many good things. If we have no way to learn about them from someone we trust, we may shrug and miss out on something good. I took my youngest son, then a teenager, some twenty miles out of town to a lovely farm and a teacher I will never forget.

Our Monday evenings with Judy and the class were challenging, though not strenuous. I stretched and strengthened, did forward bends, standing poses and the rest she thought beginners should attempt. I learned a hand stand I could manage by posing in a doorway where I could put my back against one door jam and walk my feet up the other before kicking upright. For the first time in years I felt connected to my body. I felt like I had some control.

Then, there is something about putting the body in good form that relaxes and smoothes out the mind. So I got benefits at both levels. I could use lessons I learned in yoga class to guide me in the rest of my life as well. In class and in practice I had to be persistent and steady, willing to be in a reasonable amount of discomfort and, at the same time, careful not to ask more of the body than it could do. It was the same in life. I found I could put my mind in discomfort for the sake of looking in new places—without straining to believe anything that went against my own sense of truth.

I have continued a limited practice, neither time-consuming nor strenuous but enough to keep flexible. Today I can lift my leg and set my foot on a table, though I don't show off in the community room. There are few seniors who could do it. Yoga was a great and lasting gift.

Five Issues. When I was in my mid-sixties I consulted an MD who was also trained in alternative medicine. She gave me several diagnoses: Candida, hypothyroidism, permeable intestine (leaky gut), hypoglycemia, and osteoporosis. In a letter she wrote to excuse me from jury duty she said the prognosis for significant improvement was limited. Not that I was noticeably ill. I hiked miles in a nearby state park, yet I could not have sat as a juror without excusing myself to pee and snack.

She gave me a program to follow for each disorder, including a natural thyroid medication. I needed much less of it than she thought I would and before long I didn't need it at all. When it comes to medicine, I make getting off it a priority. But I kept thinking about her letter and vowed to improve. I told myself that she put it strongly so that I would have a permanent exemption from jury duty— and she was right there. Still, I promised myself *significant improvement.*

A body's condition results from a combination of physical endowment and the habits and thoughts of the person. Ideally, the personality is stronger. As I mentioned earlier, within a few years I had resolved three of these five issues. For more than two years I went without sugars until yeast was no longer overgrown in my tum and body. The thyroid had found balance and was working optimally on its own. And I had reduced gut leaking.

That left osteoporosis, and I knew the best protection for fragile bones was to keep the muscles strong. To have good balance. I kept up the yoga, which is, among other things a weight-lifting practice since each posture carries the weight of part or all of the body. And always I kept walking and hiking.

But there were a couple problems this doctor did not find.

2017. For a number of years I have taken potassium every day and, in the heat of the summer, sea salt tabs. Now I take an electrolyte mix that covers it all. Without electrolytes the body cannot live. And if your body doesn't hang onto them well even when you eat plenty of fruits and vegetables, you need supplements.

2005. Salt and the Body. Any life can have in it some close calls. When my mother was young she was playing with her siblings and cousins in a hayloft high over the floor of a barn where the grownups were husking corn. She started to slide head first off the hay toward the gape of open air. She found that wiggling even a little made her slide faster. Her younger brother saw she was in trouble and grabbed her by both feet, pulling her to safety. Her story makes me shiver—the slippery hay, the near plunge into space. I'm glad she didn't fall.

I had one close call that was only indirectly related to the childhood illness and the effects of antibiotics. When in my sixties I was trying to boost my energy, I went on a salad and water diet under the guidance of a doctor. In my push to get results, I overreached. I didn't know you could drink too much water, but I found out. Too much can reduce the saline content of the blood to the point where you can't take in any more water, not a drop. I spent the night on the couch, too sick to get up and go to bed. When I went to the bathroom toward morning, I walked in a curled posture to protect my core. IV saline at the ER saved me. The doctor said I could have had a seizure or a heart attack. He looked up the herbs I had taken in a drink and thought one of them might have been the cause. But I was skeptical. Later a friend told me about the danger of drinking too much water. Scary. But I guess I shouldn't feel alone in my ignorance. The doctors didn't know either—or they didn't guess I would have done that. They kept me overnight and the next day until my saline measure and blood pressure came up to suit them. As to the latter, I didn't know what all the fuss was about. I was so used to low blood pressure it felt normal. At that time no one looked into the other electrolytes beyond salt, which are potassium, calcium, and magnesium.

The experience taught me moderation, even in the pursuit of health.

2017. I wake up thinking it's time to call my daughter-in-law and ask how my grandson is doing. He has his own tummy story. He and I understand each other.

Infant at Risk, 2009. People often don't realize the damage antibiotics can do to the ecology of the digestive track. My son and his wife learned too late that when she had to take antibiotics for an infection immediately after childbirth, she should not have nursed the infant. They didn't know for several years that antibiotics had come through the breast milk and wiped out most of his good gut bacteria. He was a baby who tended to throw up half of what he drank and a little boy who complained of tummy aches. My grandson was lucky, though. His parents figured out the root of his troubles and started him on a limited diet of food he could tolerate while supplementing with probiotics. In the last four or five years he has been able to add many foods back into his diet without tummy distress.

2017. My medicine cabinet holds homeopathic preparations, eye drops for allergies, some doxycycline in case of a tick bite, a bottle of Tylenol I rarely use, Bandaids, Gax-X, and Benedryl, which I keep in case of serious itching from allergies—and hope not to need. An array of supplements takes up space in my kitchen cupboard. Most are suggested by alternative doctors and muscle tested for compatibility with my body.

The Health Spa, 2012 to 2017. When I moved to my present home and set my apartment up as a research center and healing kitchen, I consulted a variety of health professionals I have come to trust, most of them within driving distance and one I talk with by email. My computer is always handy for finding health information and treatments, though I use it carefully.

I tell myself to walk, to rest, to eat, to take supplements, and I obey. I buy vegetables from local markets, make salads and soups and broths—and I sit myself down to eat and drink.

By the time I opened my personal spa, much health news was shared on the internet, with video lessons available from reliable doctors and information about herbal, homeopathic, and other holistic medicines. One of the Naturopathic doctors I consulted was a friend of my boys from their teen years—I'm proud of him for what he accomplished as part of the movement back to natural medicine.

At first I felt put-upon having to do for myself, but paying others to do all the thinking and providing would be a cop out. I wouldn't even know for sure that they were doing the right thing. I wanted to be responsible for my care and I wanted to make my own decisions, in consultation with my doctors.

Often I had a, um, gut feeling about what was wrong and what was not. For example, one doctor misdiagnosed the cause of bloating and burping as reflux and gave me a medication to reduce stomach acid, which seemed strange. Maybe I didn't have *enough* stomach acid, I argued. Seniors are apt to need more, not less. He wasn't interested in my opinion. Instead of taking the prescription, I increased my intake of organic apple cider vinegar and got some relief. I decided, wrongly as I found, that the yeast problem had returned. Put myself on a regimen of yeast control, trying several supplements and getting some relief from each, though the problem was still there when I stopped. I needed a deeper answer—but I did not need prescription medicine for a disease I did not have.

Lesson. Beware of any doctor who cannot tolerate a patient's opinions and guesses. Patients may not be doctors, but they live intimately with one body, while the doctor only reviews the information that presents in a ten minute session, and he does that according to his own flow chart. If your doctor refuses to listen to you, he may lack confidence in himself. And what is a person with such a tender self-confidence doing in a healing profession? We need doctors who appreciate our input and let us be co-responsible for our health.

We should always be ready to get ourselves out of trouble, either single-handedly or in consultation with others. It never pays to wait to be rescued.

Working as a nanny one winter, I learned a lesson in saving oneself. The toddler I was caring for lived with his father, his stepmother, and his newborn brother on the second and third floors of the house. The first floor was rented out. One afternoon I went up to the third floor to get the baby up from his nap.

I lifted him out of the crib and set him on his feet. He ran to the bedroom door and slammed it shut. I'd seen many a toddler delight in opening and shutting doors so this didn't bother me—until I tried to open the door and found it locked. From the outside. The boy's father had turned the lock around because he didn't want the child to be able to lock and unlock it from the inside. But I hadn't been forewarned.

I hadn't brought my cell phone upstairs with me. At first I tried to get the stepmother's attention by banging on the floor. I banged loud but she didn't respond. She thought the downstairs tenant was doing carpentry. By now the toddler was crying. He needed his diaper changed and he was hungry. I sat down on the floor and tried to hold him but he twisted away and cried at the door. I thought, I hope someone finds us before I need to pee.

I did have my wallet in my pocket, and I had heard of using a credit card to jimmy a lock. I thought, a real heroine doesn't sit around waiting to be saved. She saves herself and the child. I got up. The little boy looked at me and stopped crying. I took out a credit card, said to the baby "here goes" and slid the card down past the lock. It moved. The door opened.

And the incident was over—just like that.

The *save yourself* attitude got me through any number of problems. I wasn't smug about it either. It was a matter of survival.

Healing at my personal spa was like taking off in a jet plane, slowly at first and then faster

and faster until in the past several months this
health journey has lifted off into the skies.

2017. We seniors like to keep a puzzle going on one of the large tables in the community room. On Bingo night I often go work on the current puzzle and listen to the banter. They hear a number called and tease about someone's birth year. If one person wins two games in a row, someone asks, "Don't you have something to do in your apartment?" That gets a laugh. At break they serve soda and cookies or a cake, maybe a pie—sugar and wheat. I leave the puzzle table and visit friends while they snack. They say, "How can you sit with us and never eat dessert?" I say, "It isn't willpower. It's the pain." They laugh.

What Should We Eat? 1950 to 2017. Food is a strong part of any healing program. In the sixties and seventies there were lots of books on diet, including most famously Frances Moore Lappe's *Diet for a Small Planet* (1971), based on the idea that eating only vegetables would make our food resources easier to share. Coming as it did in reaction to industry meat, the book caught on rapidly. Fast forward to *The Vegetarian Myth* (2009) by Lierre Keith and that

98

idea is refuted, at least to my satisfaction. Keith demonstrates that all life is intimately linked in mutual survival. For example, apple trees feed on the bones of animals. To avoid chemical fertilizers, vegetable gardens need animal manure.

Well, maybe it's okay to eat meat—just not industry meat.

There were protein diets and carb diets and all sorts of well-meaning nonsense that never touched my parents but set my generation in a whirl. I call it nonsense because it was all so self-conscious, not the diet of a people who knew themselves.

The 1980s diet advice that made the most sense to me was to stay away from processed foods. I stopped eating white sugar and ground our own wheat flour.

In 2004 I discovered from Dr. Peter D'Adamo's *Eat for your Blood Type* that my northern European ancestors had been eating meat for centuries. In the north temperate zones, for the winter months, meat was often the only food available. During the seventies and eighties I became a vegetarian on the "when in Rome" principle. I lived among vegans, many with carb burning bodies, happy with a diet of beans and wheat, especially with plenty of vegetables and fruits. But part of me was starving and I knew it. What a relief to add animal protein and fats back into my diet and to skip grains. I could not digest grains and beans, the basic combination in Lappe's complete proteins. I needed butter on my green beans, not margarine, and I needed eggs.

When my daughter-in-law introduced me to eating Paleo, I hardly had to change, having come to it on my own. It was a diet that nourished me and made basic good sense, especially to one who had read about the origins of agriculture and animal husbandry as the root of many of our present problems.

Most recently I have tweaked my food choices along the lines of Dr. Berg's book *The Seven Principles of Fat Burning,* an easy adjustment from Paleo eating. The purpose is to get your body burning fats for fuel, something I had been doing for more than a decade, best I could. That is, I burned the fats I ate, but I did not burn stored fat.

Ideally I'm a locavore—one who eats food grown locally. I admire the macrobiotic tenet that our bodies and our food belong to the region where we live. Each area has its own soil unlike any other. No doubt a good part of my health today comes from eating the very nutritious fresh vegetables and grass-fed meat grown locally.

Local farms are our future. These smart, diverse farms with their rotation methods are rapidly replacing topsoil that has been lost in the last century. Buying locally makes economic sense, too. A farm is a local business. The dollars you spend on their products stay in the area.

2017. During other winters I have had trouble with dust and mold in my apartment. This winter, no reactions. It's nice to be free of the bouts of itching and runny nose—and I don't need to buy homeopathic allergy sublinguals at the rate of previous winters.

Allergies and Acupuncture, 2015. In my role as provider, I consulted with friends and scoured the internet in order to understand the way an allergy works. What goes wrong when you have an allergic reaction to something other people seem to tolerate?

Dr. Avery Jenkins, a practitioner of Chinese medicine, a nutrition consultant, chiropractor, and my chief health consultant, reduced my reactions with acupuncture treatments. I was able to stop over-the-counter allergy meds and handle the milder itches and sneezes with homeopathic allergy tabs. But I wanted to take the question deeper. And I found that the adrenal glands were responsible for regulating the immune system. The adrenals seemed to come up again and again.

2017. Once a day I put a couple of drops of peppermint oil into the water that steams in a crock pot in the living room. I don't need to buy an infuser. This does the trick. I lean over the pot for a couple minutes of breathing, getting the peppermint mist deep into my sinuses. Peppermint cleans my home air, too.

2017. Chiropractic Care, Homeopathy, Herbal Treatments and Essential Oils. When I was younger, I didn't understand the need for Chiropractic care. My ligaments were strong and my bones stayed in place well enough not to cause trouble. Now my hip-to-spine connections wander. My shoulders pull my upper back out. My neck goes out. Each of these can be painful. And no amount of twisting and turning puts these joints back in place. Monthly visits to Dr. Jenkins keep me pain free and (grin) well adjusted. Belief or disbelief don't come into it. I works.

Chiropractic and other alternative medicines were vilified in the early twentieth century. As mentioned previously, the Rockefellers were thorough in their insistence that only allopathic medicine and lab-created pharmaceutics be taught in American medical schools. Happily, Chiropractic medicine stayed clear of all this and went forward with the science and ethics of their founder, D. D. Palmer. If our parents had known that medical schools were endowed by crooks that cared not one bit about us, would they have trusted doctors with such blind innocence? It is our good fortune some MDs cannot be easily corrupted. The Ear, Nose, and Throat doctor who did my sinus surgery, Chris Loughlin, MD, once told me, "We allopathic doctors are trained to address illness and injury. If you want to be healthy, see an alternative doctor."

Homeopathy, using energy patterning, has never failed me—and to think it was all but extinguished from American medicine during the last century. I keep bottles of homeopathic pills for sleep, for sinus relief, for pain, and for gas relief. No side effects.

To these I add essential oils for aroma therapy. This may sound new-agey but, again, it works.

When I have questions I stop in at Act Natural Health in Torrington, CT. Pam Pinto, the proprietor, is educated in natural medicine and takes time to counsel her customers.

2017. After treatment for pneumonia while visiting my son, I return for aftercare to Doctor Penny, as we fondly call her. She orders a follow up x-ray to ensure my lungs are clear. She tells me, "When you come in, I know it's for something real because you take care of yourself."

Allopathic Medicine, 2017. The difference in medical models need not be divisive as long as we stay alert and use each for what it does best. The allopathic approach to bodies saves lives. Further, the technology your MD has available for peeking inside the body is amazing, as are modern surgical procedures. Back in the 1950s surgery saved my older sister from dying of a ruptured appendix. Without a tetanus shot my brother would have died of blood poisoning after a nick from sheep shears. I mentioned earlier that IV saline once saved my life, just as penicillin did when I was a child. These are all allopathic miracles. No wonder my parents thought doctors were wise.

Modern medicine, with its pharmaceuticals and hospitals equipped with sterile operating rooms, has changed our culture. We no longer expect to lose our children or our loved ones at the rate we once did.

But sometimes doctors, with all they had at their disposal, couldn't help a patient. Sometimes the ones who held the secret to healing were the very ones who had been driven away or marginalized. That these are coming back is our good luck. We need all our medical practices.

And consider this. Modern medicine has ethical risks traditional medicine doesn't have. With health insurance came an incentive for doctors to keep you sick, not get you well. With prescription drug insurance, doctors became motivated to over-prescribe chemical drugs and ignore wiser treatments. I'm not convinced that many allopathic doctors believe in curing illness. They seem to believe in chemically or surgically managing disease. I had to fight to stay off dangerous medicines. I had to fight for healing, not mere management. Again and again I was driven to find alternative treatments using local alternative doctors and internet searches—taking great care before trusting what I turned up. It takes persistence to navigate in the modern medical world. Helps to have trusted friends share their experiences and resources.

The problem with MDs comes in with those who follow their training by rote without responsibility.

Before I started seeing Doctor Penny for basic health care, I had a hard time with several doctors. Allopathic doctors are good at diagnosis, if the problem is on their flow chart. And they are certainly good to have for broken bones or when surgery is unavoidable. However, in my case they missed the potassium problem. One of my first realizations after moving into the hills was that I needed to supplement potassium in order to keep my blood pressure up. I knew that potassium and salt must both be replenished in hot humid weather. The two work together, and if you are low on one, the body will try to achieve balance by spilling some of the other. Why didn't my doctor know that? He determined I was losing salt and yet he didn't consider potassium.

This was the doctor who told me I had acid reflux. Two other MDs supported his diagnosis. These doctors didn't test for all possible whys. What a muddle. I get disgusted with MDs who think the best they can do for me is to manage with drugs my slow demise.

These days, Penny, NP and Doctor of Nursing, does my physicals and tells me that my numbers on about fifty measurements are within the normal range. From the point of view of allopathic measurements, my organs and systems are sound and working well. Such information allows me to dismiss most diseases from consideration. Penny is an unusually good listener. We think things through together. She understands nutrition, has studied it on her own. When I had heart palpitations she did an EKG and sent me for a stress test. I passed both in flying colors. My heart is strong.

Reassured as to the general health of my body, I was still frustrated. Cuz what in heck was the matter?

None of my doctors are right about everything. But I have learned to trust each in the areas he or she knows best. We lost much knowledge when we dismissed or persecuted traditional healers. We are still catching up. We and our doctors must work at combining traditional wisdom with medical protocols. It takes alertness and judgment, a sort of dance of trying out a remedy to see how well it works while checking and rechecking the knowledge upon which the remedy is based. I'm willing to trust a doctor on the recommendation of friends *in a provisional way*, and see where it goes. Better health is the proof.

Meanwhile, my sister found help for a long term health problem from a chiropractor.

2017. By June it had already been a stressful seven months. My husband had gone into the hospital the previous October with multiple problems, including dementia. For me, many chores followed, from meeting with doctors to emptying the apartment and doing stacks of paperwork for the Medicaid application. In June I collapsed.

Five Doctors and the Summer of 2017. My sister stands in the kitchen holding a dust mop in one hand while gripping the back of a chair with the other. She is trying to breathe. She enjoys house cleaning but these days she has to take frequent breaks from any activity. This has been going on for several years. Her MD is treating her for asthma but the inhaler doesn't do much good. She had been forced to give up hiking because she can't walk far without stopping to breathe. There's nothing scarier than not getting enough air.

At last another sister found a chiropractor who treated breathing problems. This competent and gentle woman listened to the history of the problem and knew what to do. As our gasping sister told her of a fall while getting wood from the woodpile, one that cracked a couple ribs, and of a subsequent fall that reinjured the area, the doctor said, "You taught yourself to take shallow breaths to avoid the pain, and you breathed like that over a period of months because of the second injury." The doctor knew how to release muscles that had seized up and how to guide her back to deeper breathing. Last time I checked in with her, she and her husband were out on the trails again.

That's the first doctor.

The next four each provided crucial information and care that turned a very bad summer around for me.

I thought my last days were upon me. You know, perhaps, of the man who was sitting in church one Sunday morning when the preacher asked how many wanted to go to heaven. Seemed everyone stood up except one guy. The preacher looked at him. "Don't you want to go to heaven?" "Sure. But I thought you were getting up a load to go today."

I'm with him.

My neighbor, age ninety-seven, was worried about the smell of exhaust in our hallway. She said, "I sleep with the windows open. I'm not afraid to die but I'm very fussy about *how* I die."

She speaks for me. I don't want to die in some silly, avoidable way. *And I don't want to die in confusion. Before I die I want to know what in tarnation goes on with this body.*

I count as the first of my four doctors of the summer of 2017 the Nurse Practitioner I mentioned above, who told me all my numbers were good and my heart was strong. When I have a health question to solve, I like to start with those basic allopathic measurements, the ones they get from analyzing your blood and pee. Those were all fine.

I started getting dizzy or light-headed in early June. Sometimes it felt like vertigo, which I had not experienced since I was pregnant with Ben. At the end of May I noticed my balance seemed to be off. I stumbled twice on a set of shallow stone steps. Along with the light-headedness, I started to feel really low energy and sick all over, though not with any cold or flu or such. Felt like I was six years old again and toxic because my kidneys weren't working. When I went to bed at night my heart felt like it was jumping out of my chest. As well, my tummy was always unhappy.

A friend drove me to see Dr. Jenkins. He suggested a test that showed a bacterial pathogen in my digestive tract. The testers said I seemed to have had it for some time "judging by the poor condition of the intestinal immune system." Those were the bugs causing the bloating and burps. I didn't have yeast. I really had licked it some years ago when I thought I had. I had been pretty sure I didn't have acid reflux and I didn't know any other explanation so I believed it was yeast. Nope. Bacteria. The lab tested for treatment and told my doctor what herb the pathogen would not like. He gave me a tincture and I have been gradually healing. Note that in nature there are no bad microbes. They are the cleanup crew, part of the cycle of life and death. It is in civilization we get things out of balance. I tell the pathogen, "It's not time for cleanup. So scram."

Backing up a bit, not knowing about the pathogen yet because it took a few weeks to get the results, a friend suggested I look up Dr. Eric Berg on the internet. She followed his books and videos and used some of his supplements such as electrolytes and wheat grass. I answered a long questionnaire and got a coach who worked closely with the doctor. *They determined low adrenal function as my primary problem.* No surprise. Dr. Caprile, NRT, had said the same. I have no doubt that the whole food supplements Dr. Caprile gave me for adrenal support kept disaster at bay—until this difficult year. The adrenals are in charge of balance and the distribution of hormones, enzymes and minerals. A prolonged period of stress will get the adrenals unhappy because they are the first responders to trouble. Dr.

Berg suggested electrolytes and lots of rest. (Electrolytes are mostly potassium with some salt, calcium, and magnesium.) I read his books and watched his videos on YouTube. Other supplements from Dr. Berg included an adrenal support, a gallbladder support, Vit D3 and Vit K2. With an electrolytes powder that stirred into water, lightheadedness went away over night. So did the fluttery feeling in the top of my chest. And if these symptoms came back all I had to do was take electrolytes to make them disappear. Magic.

This was making sense to me. After seven months spent getting my ex-husband into dementia care and handling his affairs, for "vacation" I spent the month of March helping my busy son and his wife. Both working at full time jobs, they urgently needed me to help with the children while their usual help was away. I drove the five hours to their home on a pleasant day. Next day we had a 20" blizzard. Three children stood at the glass door watching Papa shovel snow, bemoaning the fact that their snowsuits were all at school. We all ended up with colds and, mentioned above, I got a throat infection that went into pneumonia, first time in my life. Doxycycline, two rounds, cleared my throat and lungs but gave my digestion a set-back.

So yes, leading up to the June dizziness and feelings of toxicity I had had a bit of stress.

In June, the potassium pulled me out of one kind of lousy and the tincture cut back the burping distress I'd had had for at least four years and likely longer. I started to have some good days, and on those days I got things done and thought about the future. But I still had crummy days. Sometimes it was all I could do to stand up at the grocery store long enough to buy food.

Something wasn't right. I consulted my NRT doc, found I had an old scar that was preventing healing because some of the nerves in the skin had been cut. He treated me for that. With the scar healed I started responding to the other treatments. He told me of a girl he had helped who had a withered left wrist the doctors could not seem to cure. He noticed she had an earring through the cartilage of the right ear, looked up the meridians—sure enough, that spot controlled the left wrist. Treatment to the ear healed the wrist. I had had success with healing a scar in the past so this was not entirely new to me. The skin is an amazing organ and those nerves that run at the surface can be interfered with.

By now I had four docs. I could not have put this puzzle together without all four. Seemed like I was home free.

But wait. Something's still not right.

I'm walking back and forth in my apartment feeling too sick to lie down, walking and puzzling. I'm doing everything right, taking the tincture, drinking electrolytes, eating right, walking each morning. I'm not lightheaded, yet I go to bed feeling crappy. I fall asleep telling myself, Feels like I'm toxic with something, but what? Makes no sense. I do not feel worse overnight. In the morning I feel fine. But why? What had been so wrong yesterday and lifted completely by morning?

It comes to me that just as there is yeast die-off when you treat Candida, there may well be bacteria die-off. Sure did feel the same. With my vivid memories of that long ago Thanksgiving, I knew what it felt like to be toxic. Heck, I didn't have to remember back that far, having recently suffered the metal toxins. Now, in 2017, I realized I had felt worse since starting the tincture. Wow! I was toxic because the treatment *was working.* That meant I could moderate the intensity by taking the treatment more slowly.

It all came together. I reduced the amount of tincture I was taking and found the sweet spot where it helped me enough without the die-off making me sick. There is nothing like toxicity to make you feel like you are dying. It's awful. I'm glad I'm out of it and no longer checking to make sure my affairs are in order. As before, I regulated potassium intake to keep good balance, to keep a clear head, and to settle heart palpitations.

All this had taken a lot of thinking.

My sister's comment when I told her about my summer was that there are resources out there but *you have to integrate them.*

2017. For me, problem solving follows a pattern. First I get discouraged. My body feels sick and I can't think of anything further I can do to help it. I think, maybe this is the end of the line. I can't find a way through. Yet I don't feel ready to give up. I go to sleep in a quandary, looking from every angle. What have I missed? Is there an option I haven't thought of? I wake in the morning with a new idea, a way to go forward.

The Biggest Ahah! 2017. To recap, by the end of the summer I had handled the lightheadedness and learned that potassium is essential to every body function. No wonder I had felt so deeply sick. Every cell and system had been crying for help, either from low glucose or from low potassium or from toxicity. I still needed to eat often, though seriously low glucose moments were fewer. NRT had uncovered a bladder infection and treated it homeopathically. Acupuncture had settled the pesky environmental allergies to a level I could handle with homeopathic sublinguals. Dr. Jenkins was successfully treating me for the bad bugs that had long resided in my tummy. I was taking probiotics regularly. I also made sure to eat fermented vegetables and unsweetened yogurt.

The effort was not to get rid of one unhelpful strain of bacteria but to run a robust digestive system where one bad guy can easily be kept in line. My doctor likes to say that in the intestine there is "only so much real estate." Probiotics settle the good guys there in numbers.

I read Dr. Berg's book about the adrenals.

One evening I went to bed thinking about my long history of troubles, that two-branched legacy of tummy woes and poor stamina, both of which had their deepest roots in infancy and childhood illness. In the wee hours of the morning I woke up with the thought that perhaps my adrenals had been somehow compromised at the same time as my kidneys. Perhaps they too had been infected—and, unlike the kidneys, never completely healed. My theory wasn't accurate, but it was close. And low adrenal function dating back to age six would explain an awful lot. Might not make it possible to heal completely—the damage happened a long time ago—but knowing what had happened to my health and energy back then and through the years was *oh my goodness* satisfying. I lay in bed savoring the moment. I told myself, I think I've got it. I've got the whole picture now. I may have fetched this theory from far over the hills or maybe it had been handy as my dinner fork, but it was highly plausible and explained much. I decided to look up the adrenal glands. Wikipedia told me these glands "help in the regulation of blood pressure and electrolyte balance." Since that is not a completely reliable site, I checked further. A site called Your Hormones said the adrenal glands help "to maintain the body's salt and water levels which, in turn, regulates blood pressure." I knew that I had been able to raise my blood pressure with potassium. And I knew that adrenaline helps the body spring into action under stress and that chronic stress will cause seeping from the adrenals and lead to the exhaustion of adrenal hormones. I figured I had had plenty of stress in my life, and I could see it had been circular, the low functioning of the adrenals causing crises that had to be met by, ironically, the adrenals. In my case, those little glands that sit atop the kidneys must have been heroic. From time to time I give my body a thank you pat.

The adrenal light blazed. I knew so much now. Take this thought. I could die any time. My death certificate could give the cause of death as a heart attack. But the cause behind the heart attack could well be low potassium.

The heart can't function without sufficient potassium. And the cause of low potassium might be the inability of stunted adrenal glands to regulate and balance the body's electrolytes, of which potassium is the largest portion. The cause of damaged adrenals was the illness at age six and the stress of having an adamant mother. The cause of the illness was a system weakened by the doses of Karo syrup in infancy.

Oh, heck. Let's say the cause of my death is my birth. As I was realize soon, not all births are equal.

Following the possible causes back through the years was exuberant fun. My mental scan saw one mystery after another fall: dark circles under my eyes, poor stamina during grade school, lack of vitality for hiking, inability to do my share, disruption of the thyroid and endocrine system, which the adrenals monitor. Allergies and bug bites itchier by the year because the adrenals could no longer do the immune stuff they had done. The list wouldn't stop.

A friend once remarked that I didn't know how to shift into stress energies. In situations where other people would make that shift, carry on through, and rest later, I would fold. Now I understood. The adrenals are in charge of that shift into high gear—and mine couldn't shift.

I once saw my mother make that shift. One summer at the end of a long trip to the Rockies and back to Maine, we crossed the state line into New Hampshire at dusk. Dad was driving and Mom was looking for a motel where we could spend the night before heading home in the morning. She said she was exhausted and she did sound tired. But we hit a stretch with no motels. Dad drove on and Mom found nothing. After an hour she said, "Let's head for home. I'll take the wheel." She squared her shoulders and drove three hours, pulling into our dooryard after eleven in the evening. Said, "You kids brush your teeth and go to bed. We'll unpack the car in the morning." Sounded cheerful and energetic. Now I understood how she had done it. Suddenly I also understood the women in community households—how they had stood on their feet and worked on through fourteen-hour days.

When I was pregnant with my youngest and had a toddler and a five-year-old to tend, our family lived in a household of forty. That meant forty people to feed each evening from scratch with no refrigeration. Lots of dishes to wash, lots of pots and pans, no dishwasher except human hands. The task was daunting even for people of normal energies. It was decided that five couples would each take a weekday evening, while the single folks would divide the weekend evenings. Wednesday was our evening. After putting the children to bed, instead of gratefully falling asleep, I hauled myself back downstairs, drew a pan of soapy water, and began on the cups and plates. My husband finished a late dinner and rolled up his sleeves to help, not minding the chore. He quipped, "When Rita cooks she uses every pot in the kitchen and leaves flour in the silverware drawer." I was exhausted to the point of tears. And I knew the next day was already in ruins.

But our system was fair. On what grounds could I complain? I blamed myself for not being a good enough voluntary peasant, which was one of the ways we saw ourselves. If I complained, the others would surely think I was not a bodhisattva, *one who vows to save all beings*.

Now, after four decades, my illness was visible at last and I could give it a name: adrenal fatigue, possibly irremediable.

What a relief to know that the deficiency had been in my body, not in my willingness. I had been a faithful bodhisattva after all. I had done my best. It is hard to live with a hidden disease. Now at last it was out in the light. Nor can I blame any of the people who thought I wasn't doing my best. None of us knew.

This tummy story is long and now includes, by surprise, the second branch of trouble started in infancy, one beyond the tummy and yet interwoven with it, the adrenal story.

Why didn't I think of the adrenals sooner?

For one thing, Dr. Caprile with Nutrition Response Testing and appropriate whole food supplements had kept me in fairly good tone. I had never told him the history. But why didn't any of my other doctors, even the ones who helped me the most, think of the adrenals? I know why. I'm the only one who could view the whole pattern. I lived the life and knew the mysteries. Now I watched those mysteries tumble like the dominoes we children stood in long curving lines on the living room floor. When we were ready we tipped the end domino which hit the next and so on with a satisfying rush of clicks along the straight stretches and around the curves until all the dominoes were felled.

Click. Why all medicines seemed to make me sick. Why a natural supplement taken early in the day would still be in my system at bedtime. Why during college a sugary coke in the early afternoon would keep me awake until three in the morning. The adrenals supervise the processing and balancing. Click. A trip hiking up Mt. Tam north of San Francisco when I couldn't keep up with my pregnant sister-in-law, much less my husband and teenage sons. My brother-in-law hung back to keep me company while the rest trooped ahead. As I explained to him, "I have hit an absolute ceiling and cannot push beyond it."

Click. The night I yelled at Ben. Click. Driving up Franklin Mountain at midnight exhausted after having risen at dawn with my chirping toddlers. Click. Pulling myself up that steep place on East Rock and shaking for hours afterwards.

Compromised adrenal glands, together with toxicity and bouts of low glucose, explained every agonizing hour. I had known it in my, uh, tummy, in the center where, among other organs, the adrenals sit creating hormones critical to life.

Dominoes kept falling. Becoming toxic with three different metals during my sixties? Do adrenals play a part in detoxification? There was an flood of satisfaction, of vindication even, for each and every such memory. I could now look upon myself as a person of integrity, the person I knew I had been all along.

Another domino tips as I write the last bits of the story. A glucose domino. Please bear with me. This story begs to be told even in the closing chapters. When I was three I sometimes fainted—I have just now remembered. The last time I fainted I was standing beside my mother, my toddler sister on her lap. Wishing for help, I watched the wood floor of the Grange hall softy come up to meet me. When I came to, lying on a settee, Mother told me, "You do that again and I'll pick you up and drop your head down!" I took that to mean she'd let my head bang on the floor. After that I was too frightened to faint, giving me extra adrenalin, I guess, to stay upright. Since I never fainted again, she was sure I'd done it on purpose. I hadn't. But how can a child explain? Could those faints have been from low glucose? It keeps coming back to corn glucose from six weeks on and the thought that my body had never learned to pull energy from stored food. My immature adrenal glands must have been taxed by fear before the kidney infection.

In later years Mom said, "Oh, no. I never meant I would let your head hit the floor. Putting your head down would have been the right thing to do." Remember what I said about rehabilitating my own powers of observation. I remembered clearly the angry threat and *I know she meant to scare me.* One of my mother's chief goals was to have her children under her control. Another was to never, ever be wrong. She wasn't strong enough to apologize. In the world of my childhood, adults mostly didn't. As to that, in many families today you can still observe children taking the blame for what the parents do.

There is a rightness to my mother's posture. Deep down we know we are good, and we believe we cannot have done wrong. It is important not to blame individual parents for the mistakes they make. The mistakes are in the culture.

What if Mom had not been alone on a hill farm far from other women and the neighborly help women give one another? What if she had known that nursing her first daughter longer would have put enough space between pregnancies for her body to regain strength to support the next baby? What if her own parents had not hurt her, giving her a way to grow her own confidence? What if she had seen a child's faint as a physical event, not the action of a bad child?

Getting back to the adrenals, I checked my theory with Dr. Jenkins. He thought it would not have been infection but immature adrenals stressed to where they never completely recovered. I asked him also about my infancy. I told him, "My sister was only fourteen months old when I was born. I wonder whether my mother's body was not ready to support a second baby so soon." (My mother knew nothing of birth control. And I expect she was eager to give her husband a son.) I told the doctor the born skinny and screaming story and the solution of cow's milk with Karo syrup.

He said, "I can see exactly what happened. An infant's digestive tract does not come already populated with microbes. It gets some on the way through the birth canal and the rest from nursing." He said my mother's milk may have lacked the needed microbes. "Was the cow's milk raw?"

"Yes. It would have been. My father kept a cow to milk for the family."

"That's why you stopped crying." Raw cow's milk would have supplied the microbes.

All the mysteries were solved.

2017. I came close to never knowing what really happened. Solving the story required living to gather all the facts. I was stubborn. I refused to die until I knew. I'd done my best to eat nutritious food. And I was lucky in meeting friends who knew good resources.

Triumph, 2017.   The information and guidance I have gathered about how to survive and live well suggests that we as a people have work to do: to grow food at or near home, to outlive the diseases that have been with us since we crowded up in cities where sewage ran in the streets, and to outlive modern disorders that come from eating non foods and from taking lots of prescription drugs and antibiotics. The age of antibiotics is coming to a close. We need to grow our bodies strong and care for them in healing ways that do not bring further trouble, judiciously using all the healing models that work.

A number of books and documentaries urge us to restore pasturelands and the tall prairie grasses that once supported healthy bison and antelope with soil many feet deep, now mostly washed away. As Sir Albert Howard said many years ago, "The health of soil, plant, animal, and man is one and indivisible." (see IFOAM Organics International webpage)

In these actions rests our triumph over sore tummies and the disruptions of the endocrine system that come with the stress of disease.

When my siblings and I were kids we used to make up Tom Swifties. One sister came out with one I love to recall. "Umph! Umph! Umph! she said triumphantly."

Triumph is what I feel now—and what I want to feel for all of us. Umph enough to see my dreams through, dreams that involved a lot more than figuring out what was wrong with one body. The tummy story was always a side story, not the point of living. For me, a life should be full of family and friends and satisfying projects.

I may not be able to bring my adrenals into normal range of functioning. But with electrolyte supplements and other measures of comfort and support, I can continue to coax these valiant little glands, so indispensible to life, to continue to partner with me a while longer. I can visit grandchildren and write stories for their birthdays. I can write and publish my work, each book a part of a wide conversation about health and life, our history and the promise of our future. I can enjoy the social life where I live. I've made it to a graceful old age and that is a win over staggering odds. I am satisfied with this life and with these dominoes lying on their backs open to be read. It's a triumph.

What I did, you can do, too. I will cheer.

I know what I want at my memorial service. Leonard Cohen singing his hauntingly beautiful "Hallelujah." Someday.

And that's the tummy story that started with the first bottle of cow's milk my mother gave me in caring innocence, not guessing that the milk would populate my tummy with helpful bugs and let me sleep and grow into a life.

She liked me better when I smiled.

I thought when I wrote the first edition of Tummy Story I was writing something widely experienced. And I suppose I was speaking for many when I suggested methods of consulting health practitioners and doing research. But I have realized that the particulars of my story are not common. Rarely have I met anyone who experienced hypoglycemia starting in infancy. I don't know of anyone whose adrenals were stunted from a childhood illness, though I feel sure it has happened to others. The trouble I have had with digestion is a little more common, I think, but none of the seniors who live in this building of thirty-six apartments has mentioned tummy woes; presumably they do not have an over-abundance of the bad bacteria that annoys and interrupts my life and has for many years.

Among the many lessons I've learned while writing and revising this book it that my story is a bit peculiar. Not only is it unusual, but the final piece only fell into place after I was 78 years old. In this tale the final insight is the first, the one that set all the rest in motion.

A quick review would go like this:

a) My mother was an undernourished teenager during the Great Depression of the 1930s, a time when their family meals were either oatmeal or cornmeal mush.

b) Her body was not ready for a second pregnancy a few months after the first.

c) I was born malnourished.

d) Breastfeeding didn't work for us because her milk lacked the probiotics natural to mother's milk.

e) An infant that screams for six weeks may not get to bond well with her mother.

f) My mother's solution of giving me cow's milk with Karo syrup from six weeks on probably saved my life because of the probiotics in raw cow's milk. Yet the corn sugar prevented my pancreas from maturing, leading to hypoglycemia.

g) The tension between my mother and me, including spankings, made me feel rejected.

h) Rejection made me vulnerable to illness.

i) Scarlet fever at age 6 went into a bacterial kidney infection.

j) With penicillin my kidneys healed and I lived, but my adrenals apparently never recovered, giving me a lifelong lack of stamina, undiagnosed until 2017.

k) Because of penicillin my gut had to start yet again on building up an internal ecosystem.

This list of events in the history of one body adds up to a trio of lasting issues, hypoglycemia, digestive distress, and low vitality.

I now know why I have never been able to keep up, why I have always needed to carry food with me, and why my tummy hurts. I can look back through my life to a thousand instances where my lack of endurance was not the lack of willingness it seemed. Best of all, today I have a solid idea what to do, if not to reach optimum health, at least to enjoy many good hours of living. Throughout my life I have often felt I was reaching the end of my days, only to find a new way to go forward.

I have tons of information and many handlings for the various body problems that present themselves to me each day. I didn't set out to become a medical expert, and I'm not today a medical expert, but I am an expert user of one body.

And so are you. This book offers you a method that has worked for me.

This revised edition of *Tummy Story* would be incomplete without my personal list of miracles.

a) I survived prenatal malnourishment.
b) Raw cow's milk with its natural probiotics saved my life.
c) Penicillin saved my life.
d) And what a life!

e) I had three babies who become winning little boys and charming men. That's three miracles.

f) Nutrition Response Testing in the nick of time pulled me back from the brink.

g) Yoga postures introduced me to my body and strengthened me both physically and emotionally.

h) IV saline therapy in 2006 cheated death yet again.

i) All of which gave me time to write and publish more than 10 books. That's 10 more miracles.

j) Dr. Avery Jenkins' insights and treatment, including adrenal support, gave me precious information about my entire life and guidance for keeping a body on track.

k) A digestion diagnosis done by an alternative lab told me what pathogen I had and how to treat it.

l) Electrolytes have been a gift from Dr. Eric Berg, an essential one.

To put some of these miracles into perspective, without electrolyes and adrenal support, I'd be hard put to stand up or engage in any of the chores and joys of living. Add to the list a passion for life and an inclination toward detective work. Biggest miracle: against all odds I'm 78 years old. And a half, as my young grandchildren count their years.

Integrate. That was the word my sister used. Means to take responsibility for overall information and to work the various treatments together as a whole. For me this includes keeping in mind the three points of a triangle: stamina, digestion, and hypoglycemia. It includes sensing what each condition feels like when off, and which treatments can help. It means distinguishing among various body feelings, or signals, such as how low blood pressure feels (lightheaded) and how high blood pressure feels (throbbing), how low blood glucose feels (frantic, threat of imminent collapse), how toxicity feels (poisoned, sick toward death), and how low adrenaline feels (another kind of sick). Identifying each signal helps me know what to do.

People have lots of health problems, often problems far more serious than mine. But I know of few whose health requires such ongoing alertness. One friend does know what my life is like. She raised a child from toddlerhood with Type I diabetes. She said it is called "the thinking man's disease." As he grew older, her son took on the thinking—and he can never stop.

Nor can I.

2021. Here I am going along singing zip a dee do da and there's a bluebird on my shoulder and the body says, how can you be so cheerful when I'm sinking into the mud? So I stop singing and the bluebird flies away and I do my best to pull the body out of the mud, throw a bucket of river water over it to clean it up. Go along again singing with the bluebird back on my shoulder and the body says, how can you be so cheerful when I'm caught in these brambles? And I stop singing and get some clippers and cut the body out of the brambles. I never can seem to get the body complcoetely out of the mud and brambles and I get tired of caring for it and tired of thinking what does it need this time. So I leave it at that and go along singing with the bluebird on my shoulder and the whole thing happens all over again. I used to have a lot of affinity for this body, mostly still do. But I can't help dreaming of the day I can leave it and keep the bluebird.

Acknowledgements

My tummy and I are deeply grateful to the following doctors and friends for guidance and good cheer, as well as for truth in an age of hidden dangers to our health. Avery Jenkins, DC, DCBCN, FIAMA. Well-educated in the healing arts, Dr. Jenkins is an exceptionally good listener, able to fit together seemingly unrelated data. As well, through chiropractic adjustments he keeps my bones in place. Bob Caprile, DC, practitioner of Nutrition Response Testing, and Freddie Ulan, DC, creator and teacher of Nutrition Response Testing. These wonderful doctors are gentle and acutely aware of health issues. Without Freddie and the doctors he has trained I might not have lived into my sixties and would certainly not have known about the scars and metal toxicities that blocked healing. Robert Scarszynski, DC, who, in addition to Nutrition Response Testing and treatment, rubbed adhesions out of my frozen shoulders. Dr. Adam Propper, DC, whose excellent chiropractic skills kept me pain free year after year while I lived in his area. Chris J. Loughlin, MD, ENT, whose surgery and treatment gave me back working sinuses and who understood the place of alternative medicine in any wellness plan. Penny McEvoy, DNP, APRN, ANP-BC, respectful primary care Nurse Practitioner.

Edyth Mercier, dear friend and guide through many a health crisis. Rob Carr, beloved friend and writer as well as font of health resources and good natural stuff to keep in the medicine cabinet.

Act Natural Health and Wellness in Torrington, where Pam Pinto, the proprietor, is generous with her time and education, became a great resource. Thanks, Pam.

Robin Rose, MD, my North Star and long time friend, gave me what guidance she could from far away, guidance grounded in both science and nature. Dr. Robin, as we fondly call her, inspires both trust and affection.

Bibliography

A Basic Call to Consciousness: The Hau de no sau nee Address to the Western World. Presented in Geneva, Switzerland, 1977. Copyright 1978 by Akwesasne Notes.

Eisler, Riane. *The Chalice and the Blade: Our History, Our Future,* HarperCollins, 1987.

Estes, Clarissa Pinkola. *Women Who Run with the Wolves, Myths and Stories of the Wild Woman Archetype,* Ballantine Books, New York, 1992.

Graf, Alan Stuart, *I Inhaled: Rantings, Ramblings and Ravings by a Hippie Lawyer.* Published by Division Books, an imprint of Di Angelo Publications, copyright 2014 Alan Stuart Graf in digital and print.

Hopkins, Rob. *The Transition Companion,* Chelsea Green, White River Junction, VT, 2011.

Keirsey, David and Marilyn Bates. *Please Understand Me: Character and Temperament Types,* Gnosology Books Ltd., Del Mar, CA, 1984.

Kingsnorth, Paul. *Real England: The Battle against the Bland,* Portobello Books Ltd, London, UK 2008.

Parkes, Henry Bamford. *The American Experience: An Interpretation of the History and Civilization of the American People,* Vintage Books, A Division of Random House, New York, 1947, 1955, 1959.

Quinn, Daniel. *Ishmael: An Adventure of the Mind and Spirit,* A Bantam-Turner Book, 1992.

Sanders, Scott Russell. *Staying Put: Making a Home in a Restless World,* Beacon Press, 1993

Sherwonit, Bill. *Animal Stories: Encounters with Alaska's Wildlife,* Alaska Northwest Books, Portland, OR, 2014.

Spence, Gerry. *From Freedom to Slavery: The Rebirth of Tyranny in America,* St. Martin's Press, 1993.

Thomas, Elizabeth Marshall. *The Animal Wife,* Houghton Mifflin Harcourt Publishing Company, New York, 1990.

Thomas, Elizabeth Marshall. *The Old Way: A Story of the First People,* Picador, New York, NY, 2006.

Books by Patricia Mitchell Lapidus, in order of publication:

Sweet Potato Suppers: A Yankee Woman Finds Salvation in a Hippie Village, published in 2003 by R S Press, Savannah, GA. Second Edition published in 2009 by Tall Woman Tales Press, now Walking Tall Tales Press.

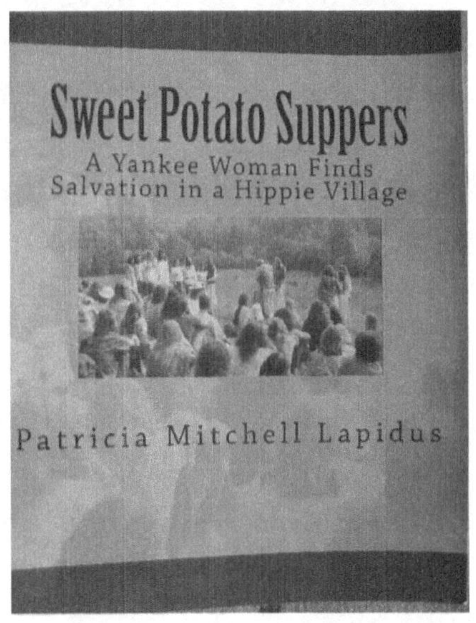

Excerpt: In the late 1970's I was declared a terrorist by the government of the United States. I was considered dangerous not in myself but in my collectivity with some 1,200 other folks, many of them children. Our family lived for almost ten years in the related communities known as The Farm, founded by Stephen Gaskin and his followers. (When in

1984 Don and I moved into town, rented an apartment, bought a car, and took jobs for wages, we were apparently no longer a threat.) How a tiny village frightened the most powerful nation on earth is one part of my story.

Sweet Potato Suppers: A Yankee Woman Finds Salvation in a Hippie Village is the story of a personal awakening from a generations' long sleep. The sleep seems to have happened like this: During centuries of trouble—war and plunder, European feudal law, famine, plague, the persecution of healers and dissidents— cruelty became a common, invisible part of the character of every woman and man. Each person experienced heart-injuring events they re-enacted blindly in daily relationships. Thus, while they made heroic efforts to benefit their children, they also frightened and scarred them.

This writing began as an apology to my children for the trouble they inherited. I wanted them to know their history, especially the deep old roots of family pain. And what The Farm, embedded in their early memories, had to do with it all. What began as an internal family message grew into this book, the story of how one family, while living in community, began reclaiming its soul.

Swamp Walking Woman, **Tall Woman Press, now Walking Tall Tales Press, 2010.**

Swamp Walking Woman is a modern, mythic fairy tale. When Swamp Walking Woman wanders into the swamp and finds a little girl asleep on a hummock, seemingly abandoned, she takes the child under her wing and looks help, finding instead a tough Gatoress who recruits her for firefly duty, which involves lighting a fire stick at the only fire allowed in the swamp and taking it across muddy water to her portion of the swamp. There the fireflies, having lost their lights because of pollution, back their rumps up to the fire stick for light.

What will it take to restore the swamp and put the powerful Gatoress in her place?

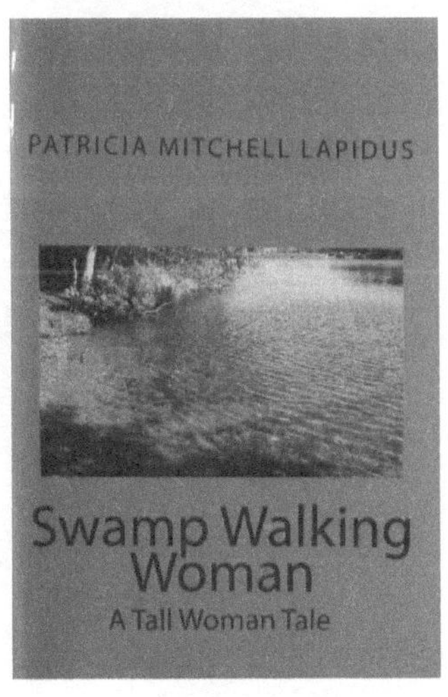

***Gideon's River,* a novel, Walking Tall Tales Press, 2010.**

Twelve-year-old Gideon has a temper, wishes he didn't have a temper, and doesn't know how not to have a temper. Gideon goes to great length to get rid of his temper and to pull some love from his absent father, who lives beyond the Catskills. Gideon's mother, watching her son get into a series of heroic troubles, learns that she can't help him until she grows her own confidence.

The novel shows how the generations tend to flip roles in the classic drama of "the bully and the wimp."

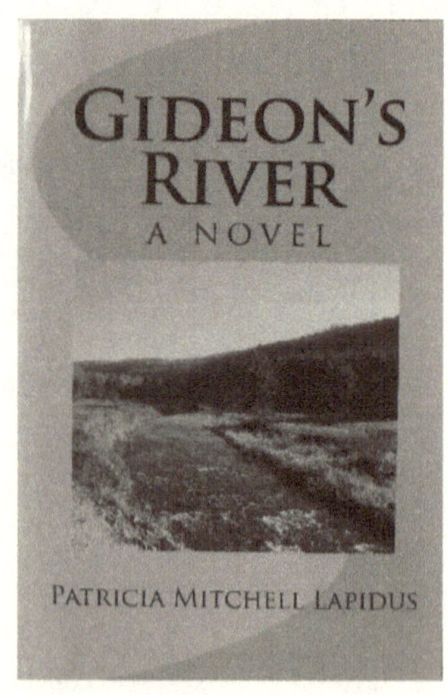

Ren Hen's Daughters, Walking Tall Tales Press, 2009 and 2017, expanded.

Many of these poems were first published in literary journals such as *Peregrine, Off the Coast,* and *Green Hills Literary Lantern.*

Song Sparrow

A song sparrow with the grace of clear purpose
feeds steadily on round millet seeds.

His precise activities and coat—
brown spot at mottled throat—hold him ho!
one whose lines will not lapse. When he
flits to the bush to begin his morning song,
a rapturous offering stronger than any I
have sung, I wonder at the size of the soul
of a bird.
       Soul, in bulkless thread, rivers
as hugely through the songbird as through me.

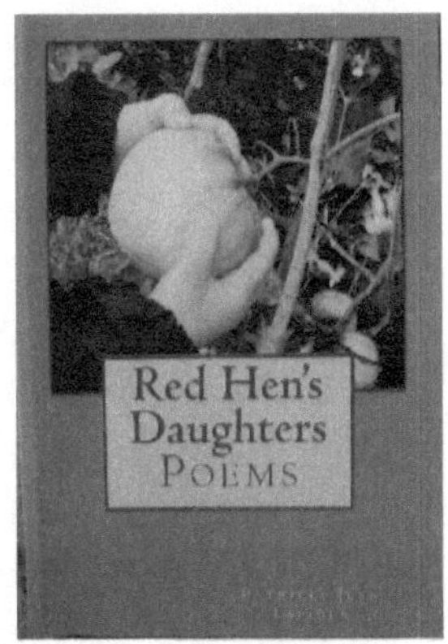

***The Farm That Tried to Feed the World:
Why Local Farms, Sharing Communities, and
Transition Neighborhoods Matter to All of Us,***
First Edition published by Outskirts Press,
2013, Second Edition published by Walking Tall
Tales Press, 2017.

The Farm That Tried to Feed the World is the
second book about The Farm, this time a
community in the Catskills that was a sister to
the one in Tennessee. *Sweet Potato Suppers*
covered five years spent on the Tennessee
Farm. *The Farm That Tried to Feed the World*
covers an additional four years of life in the
Catskill community, much of it in memoir style,
though the final chapter shifts to a recap of five
books that help an understanding of what in our
world mitigates against the sharing life.

Excerpt: On The Farm we were doing our best to
identify the unsaid and say it. We called it the
subconscious. But it was only subconscious to the
person. Anyone else could see that there was, for
example, anger disguised as tears or as criticism—and
lack of confidence below both tears and anger. That
brings us back to how and why the sort-outs worked. A
foundation belief was that someone we trusted could
give insight that could help us change bad habits and
uninspected ways of thinking. We had seen the trouble
created in the larger world by people who thought they
were being rational when they were not. It seemed

paramount to shed our baggage—and at the same time not to complain about the past but to stay in the present and give one another our goodwill, our smiles, and plenty of encouragement. Each Sunday Stephen spoke about some aspect of the wider culture we had come from, and the more transparent one we were creating with chagrin and courage and love.

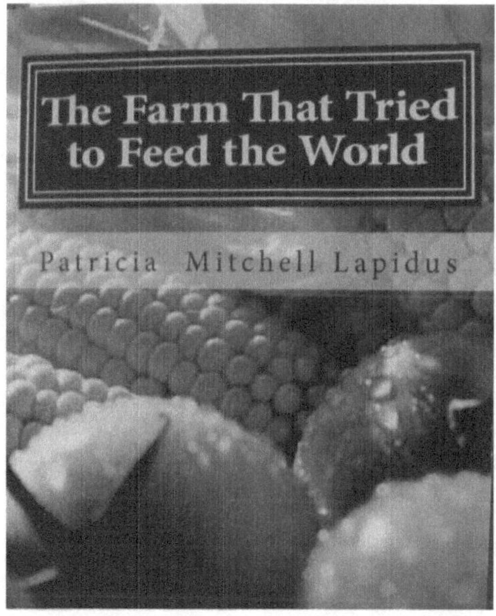

Walter Moose on Oak Hill, Walking Tall Tales Press, 2017.

Written for my grandson, in these tales a kindly and awkward moose takes the young Zachary by time travel back to the days of the boy's great-grandfather growing up on Oak Hill.

Excerpt from The Moose in the Sandbox:
"Why are you sitting in our sandbox?"
"I love sifting sand," said the moose. "Come and join me."
"I can't get in there with you. You are taking up all the room and lapping over the back."
The moose looked around at his rump. He sighed. "Can't be helped I guess, since they insist on making these things so small. Would you like to hear a story about your great-grandfather up in Maine?"
"Not particularly. I don't like old stuff and anyway I'm not going to listen to anything until you get out of the sandbox. You are not a little boy."
The moose looked himself over carefully. "No, I suppose I'm not."

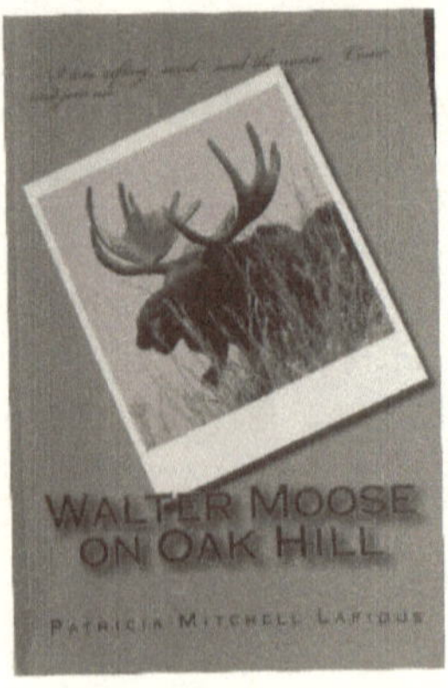